Your Guide to Health with
Foods & Herbs

Using the Wisdom of
Traditional Chinese Medicine

Zhang Yifang & Yao Yingzhi

Better Link Press

Text: Zhang Yifang, Yao Yingzhi
Photographs: Roger Yan, Zhang Yifang, Yao Yingzhi, Roy Upton, Alfred Kump, Quanjing, Ding Guoxing
Cover Image: Quanjing
Cover and Interior Design: Wang Wei

Copy Editor: Kirstin Mattson
Editor: Yang Xiaohe
Editorial Director: Zhang Yicong

ISBN: 978-1-60220-121-7

Address any comments about *Your Guide to Health with Foods & Herbs: Using the Wisdom of Traditional Chinese Medicine* to:

Better Link Press
99 Park Ave
New York, NY 10016
USA

or

Shanghai Press and Publishing Development Co., Ltd.
Floor 5, 390 Fuzhou Road, Shanghai, China (200001)
Email: sppdbook@163.com

Printed in China by Shanghai Donnelley Printing Co., Ltd.

9   1 0   8

The material in this book is provided for informational purposes only and is not intended as medical advice. The information contained in this book should not be used to diagnose or treat any illness, disorder, disease or health problem. Always consult your physician or health care provider before beginning any treatment of any illness, disorder or injury. Use of this book, advice, and information contained in this book is at the sole choice and risk of the reader.

Contents

Foreword

Traditional Chinese medicine is one of the oldest systems of healing on earth. Its power to heal lies in ancient knowledge that recognizes that human health arises from a connection to earth through one's diet, lifestyle, exercise, healing traditions and relationship to creation. The medicine plants used in Chinese as well as other traditional systems of healing connect us with this ancient knowledge and provide us with a direct link to the healing spirit of earth. Many of the botanicals originally used in Chinese medicine have now found their way into healing traditions worldwide as Chinese medical philosophy has spread. This is in recognition of the unique contribution it can make to the healing of those suffering in ways not addressed in Western approaches to health care.

This text by Drs. Zhang Yifang and Yao Yingzhi, two authorities on Chinese herbal medicine, provides a valuable contribution to the herbal medicine literature by guiding us in how we can enhance the healing power of our diet by the combining of medicinal herbs with common foods. Using herbal medicines in this way has been a common practice in Chinese culture for centuries and is often overlooked in favor of the many teas, pills, tablets and other medicinal preparations that find their way into Chinese medical practice. The highest ideal of Chinese medicine throughout the centuries has been the cultivation of principles that help us stay well rather than waiting until something is wrong and then trying to fix it. I once was told of an ancient Chinese adage, "to use herbs to treat sickness is like digging a well when you are thirsty." In other words, it is much better to incorporate medicinal plants in one's everyday life than waiting until it is too late.

This work provides unique guidance on how, on a daily basis, we can incorporate herbs into our lives to stay healthy as well as how to turn our common foods into profound medicines when we are sick. Anyone interested in the healing arts, regardless of the traditions they follow, can benefit from the experience and wisdom of these senior Chinese medical practitioners. Similarly, the knowledge and recipes contained herein can provide families with the guidance needed to bring healing practices directly into their homes in the most basic and profound way through daily nourishment. The authors are commended for sharing and expanding the knowledge of this part of Chinese healing traditions to a larger part of the world.

Roy Upton, RH, DAyu
President, Editor
American Herbal Pharmacopoeia

Preface

Finding a way to maintain a positive spirit and a healthy lifestyle has become an increasingly important focus these days. Traditional Chinese medicine (TCM), which has been relied upon by millions of people over the generations, provides simple yet effective ways to achieve optimal health through natural solutions and plant remedies. TCM can help you understand the many components that make you uniquely you! This book will enable you to put that wisdom to use, providing practical information, case studies, treatment details, recipes and illustrations.

The functional food and herbs catalogued in this book are widely available, and combine a pleasing flavor with useful medical functions. To help you find the foods that are suited to your body and lifestyle, we provide a unique self-assessment so you can learn about your individual body constitution. This, combined with remedies for common illnesses, will put you on the path to better health.

Food is a part of everyday life, so much so that you may not give it a great deal of thought. Food offers an incredible ability to heal and nourish the human body. Different foods and herbs can act like medicine in their positive effects and help sustain a healthy state over time. Since they can produce a wide range of results, and at times even harmful effects, foods should be considered and chosen carefully so as to lead to greater well-being. This attitude toward the multitude of properties that food has, and the wealth of its effects, is at the core of Chinese Medicine.

Choosing the right food is essential to getting healthy and staying that way. In making wise choices, it is important to note that some foods may be better suited to a certain person or condition than to another. We are all different, physiologically and psychologically, and foods and herbs have individualized inherent qualities as well; so we need to understand the characteristics of ourselves and our foods when making choices.

Why did I choose to focus on this topic in writing this book?

Just as the old saying goes, an ounce of prevention is worth a pound of cure. The preventative side of TCM provides an appealing and accessible point of entry to anyone who wants to learn about and use Chinese medicine. Food therapy is the easiest way to start.

Using plants for health and the prevention of illness is deeply ingrained in China's rich culture. It is an important part of my personal experience as well. My brother and I grew up in a family steeped in Chinese medical tradition; with our parents and grandparents, simple yet effective food therapy was paramount in our daily life.

When my brother and I were young, if we experienced a bout of diarrhea, our mother always told us to drink *wu mai* tea (dried dark plums boiled with brown sugar). After only one or two drinks, we would recover. As a child facing exams, I would often be nervous and unable to sleep, so my father would bring me a cup of chrysanthemum tea or some peanuts. After that, I could sleep soundly.

Those memories of simple food-based remedies stuck with me as I grew older and learned the value of the phrase, *yao bu bu ru shi bu, shi bu bu ru shen bu* (药补不如食补，食补不如神补), meaning that pharmaceutical remedies cannot compete with food remedies, which have compounded psychological effects that surpass their basic nutrient properties. *Shen bu* or psychological effects can be thought of as one's attitude toward overall wellness and total health maintenance, sometimes called the Health Quotient (HQ). By this belief, whenever doctors of Chinese medicine see a conflict between the patient's body, environment, certain foods, and/or climate, they do *not* immediately look for a prescriptive remedy. Instead, they first seek to discover the root of the conflict. Then they take steps to avoid a continuation of this conflict. Finally, they use food therapy to eliminate the conflict and balance the body.

This is a superior method of treating bodily disorders and preventing recurrence. By using food in a therapeutic way (which we term "functional foods" in this book), we are forced to listen to the body, learn about the self, and gain a greater knowledge of what the body wants and needs.

In August 1988, the day before my daughter was born, my mother handed me something and told me, "You will have a child soon. Take this bottle with you; inside is sliced ginseng that you should chew when you are in the delivery room and the contractions are getting stronger. The midwife will ask you to push and you will get strength from this ginseng to help you give birth." I did as mother instructed me and I felt strong and more able to cope with the pain of child birth. After my daughter was born, the first cup of liquid that I drank was "dragon eye" soup. For the next month, I drank a lot of soups of mixed food and herbs to nurture and restore myself.

The second reason I chose the topic of food therapy is because food is an accessible topic with universal appeal—we all eat! It has served me well in my teaching and consulting with over a million students and clients during my nearly 30 years of lecturing and clinical practice. One of my patients, Joan, did not know much about Chinese medicine, believing that TCM consisted only of painful needles and drinking bitter herbal teas. Nonetheless, she came to see me and I took the time to discover the cause of her cough, diarrhea and night sweats. The source of her condition was due to her food choices. Within ten days of using food therapy, her symptoms had disappeared and she had no more complaints.

When my family first arrived in England, we all suffered from an inability to adapt to the local environment and climate (*shui tu bu fu* 水土不服). Symptoms can include skin itchiness and blisters. As my daughter was only three years old at that time, I made an appointment for her to visit a physician to get a prescription for skin cream. After putting the cream on her hands, the rash got bigger and spread to her arms and body. I kept using the cream for a few more days, but the effect was only to make the rash worse. I decided to stop using the cream and try giving her mung bean soup, porridge and honeysuckle tea. Two days later the itchiness was reduced. In a week's time, she was better. Since then, these foods have become our family's secret skin care recipe.

Food therapy is what I discuss first when teaching or consulting with patients. After evaluating a patient's condition, what diseases they suffer from, and looking at other patterns, I tell them which foods they should avoid or eat less of, and then suggest the best foods to add to their diet.

Food can work by itself to heal, or can aid the treatment of diseases, working better than medicine alone. For example, some kinds of yoghurt can assist the function of antibiotics. Eliminating or reducing intake of certain foods can also help heal. For example, a client suffered from psoriasis, but after drinking less Chinese distilled liquor, the condition disappeared. For children suffering from eczema, reducing packaged foods, especially those with a long shelf life, will make the treatment much more effective. In this book, I will show you how to apply the magic of food, and share secret recipes to enhance your well being and your enjoyment of functional foods.

It has long been a wish of mine to share the wisdom of TCM with readers across the world. My previous book, *Using Traditional Chinese Medicine to Manage Your Emotional Health*, and this book are an attempt to realize that dream. This book seeks to integrate traditional Chinese wisdom with the fruit of modern research to create personalized solutions. TCM's natural approach to regulating and nourishing the body and mind is the most sustainable and effective way to prevent a poor quality of life and deterioration into illness over the long term.

TCM is guided by ancient philosophies that focus on opposing forces and how they are brought into balance. It seeks to understand groups of people based on shared characteristics, while at the same time, emphasizing the uniqueness of the individual. Based on the "holism" of a person, physiologically and psychologically, TCM helps bring harmony not only within a person's body, but also between people and the surrounding natural and societal environments. It emphasizes natural remedies—food and herbs—as well as adjusting the mind, before treating with medicine, because the latter is often accompanied by side effects.

Several key topics in TCM, such as Body Constitution, Yin-Yang Theory, the Five Elements, the Meridians and Organ Systems, Symptoms and Seasonal Changes, are integral to making the right food choices. In learning about these concepts, you will discover how to assess your own body constitution, how to use foods and herbs based on a range of physical and environmental factors, and how to bring balance to your daily diet.

TCM believes that food and medicine share the same source, and food can prevent and treat illness. The link between food and human health has received ever-increasing attention, as people have come to realize the truth behind the adage, "You are what you eat." You don't have to completely change your way of eating. Active awareness and easy adjustments can enhance the quality of your life and help you stay healthy.

Dr. Zhang Yifang

Acknowledgements

This book is a fruit of my research on food therapy, combining my personal experience of nearly 30 years with the knowledge and practices of traditional Chinese medicine that have developed during its 5,000-year history. Professor Yao kindly contributed her knowledge of food properties and functions (in Chapter Four) and some colorful pictures of plants.

I would like to thank both my father and father-in-law, who have always encouraged me to share my knowledge broadly, with people around the globe. I also want to thank my husband for his valuable suggestions and editing assistance.

Many thanks to my daughter, Mengyue Wu, and my friends Toffler Ann Niemuth, Amena Lee Schlaikjer and Dora Baldvinsdottir for contributing their thoughts, translation and dictation.

I would like to thank Roger Yan, a friend and a wonderful artist, who created beautiful drawings for this book and helped to bring my words to life, creating an atmosphere where art and medicine can coexist. Thanks also go to my longtime friend Roy Upton, the President and editor of American Herbal Pharmacopoeia, who wrote Foreword and generously provided some pictures of herbs for this book.

I also want to thank our editor Yang Xiaohe for her patience and support, and Kirstin Mattson for her editorial talents and logical approach.

According to the Chinese saying, *ming yi shi wei tian* (民以食 为 天), food is linked to both our body and soul. Foods bring us energy, enjoyment and happiness, and are a source of healing and defense. The approach of traditional Chinese medicine is, at its core, specific to the individual's body and needs, and therefore is of benefit to each and every person. My goal is to make TCM easy to understand, so you can put it to practice in your kitchen daily.

To use this book more efficiently and effectively, you may also want to consult my website, www.acherbs.com, and as well as my previous book *Using Traditional Chinese Medicine to Manage Your Emotional Health*.

Wish health and happiness for you and your family.

Dr. Zhang Yifang

Chapter One

General Rules for Choosing Foods and Herbs

As the traditional Chinese saying notes, "food and medicine share the same roots," which means that our daily diet not only provides nutrition and delicious flavors, but is also important for our health. In China, functional nutrition draws on thousands of years of culture, based on Chinese medicine, which recognizes that dietary regimens and herbal tonics can strengthen the body, maintain fitness, prevent disease, cure illnesses and contribute greatly to longevity and prosperity. So how can we maintain good health, and prevent and cure disease, while still enjoying delicious cuisine?

1. Taking Nationality and Culture as a Starting Point

One's diet is affected by nationality and cultural influences. We grow up and live in certain regions that influence our basic food choices. For instance, rice is a staple for Chinese people, while bread is more common in Europe and the US. Some of the foods listed in this book are international, while some are typically Chinese. Each food group has about five to eight representatives from which you can choose. It is best to start out by choosing from among those foods that are familiar to you, and building from there. Too much change from your native diet, or starting with foods you do not enjoy or are not familiar with, will only set yourself up for failure. And if you are not able to find specific Chinese ingredients, you can substitute other foods within the same family and species that can be found in your home country.

Clinical research shows that the use of food to improve one's health state may produce varied results. Generally speaking, if you are fond of something, you will do better and get more out of it. In Chinese, "being fond of" is a state of mind towards something, whether it be food therapy, or sports or other hobbies. There are two groups of people: optimistic and pessimistic. People who are fond of food in general enjoy a balanced lifestyle, take pleasure in their working environment, and are emotionally stable. It is easy then to understand that optimists tend to get better results from food therapy than the pessimistic group.

Chinese people don't deprive themselves of foods that are perhaps not always considered healthy, for example wine or fried food. They consume those items in moderation and are also mindful of using other food groups that can aid in balancing out the unhealthier ones. For instance, if you like eating sausages and luncheon meat, you should drink three cups of tea, or add vinegar to the cooking process to flush out or limit the harmful effects. Also, for those people that like to barbeque their food, they should balance it by consuming 150g of sweet potatoes first, to provide a protective layer for the stomach. Another remedy is to drink a glass of soymilk to line the stomach.

2. Considering Locality and Season

Be sure to select seasonal produce in order to get the most nutrients and health benefits. For instance, some fruits that are seasonal in the summer can assist with cooling the body. Due to globalization and technological advancements in agriculture, some food items formerly available only during the summer may now be purchased year-round. However, this disrupts the natural way and is not conducive to promoting health. Moreover, people should keep their local environment in mind. If you live in an area that is hot and humid, you need to focus on consuming food that can help reduce water retention and cool you down.

Our physical and emotional states are greatly influenced by climate and the environment, its rhythm and seasons. When we use food to assist our health, we should eat less cold food in the winter, less hot food in the summer, less spicy and pungent food in the autumn dry season and less moist food in the humid weather.

Geographical features of a place have a strong impact on both our body constitution and our food choices. People from the north can take more hot food than people who have grown up in the south. People from humid regions can tolerate wet climates better than people from dry regions.

In order to get the best quality of ingredients you should

select foods that are still produced in the area from which they traditionally originate. For instance, the best quality wolfberries come from Ningxia autonomous region and Gansu province in China. The best jujubes (red dates) are from Tianjin and Shandong province. It is advisable to always look at food packaging to see where the product originates to ensure its quality.

Additionally, it is important to keep in mind that you can consume larger quantities of fresh produce as opposed to dried. Dried produce is more potent and causes stronger reactions in the body.

3. Balancing the Five Flavors

Chinese medicine categorizes food into five basic flavors—salty, sweet, sour, spicy and bitter. Each flavor has a special function and health benefit.

For example, different nationalities may consume different foods when facing stress and daily pressures. In China, this tends to be more jujubes and bananas; in the US and Europe, this tends to be more chocolate and cookies. However the tastes are the same: sweet and spicy. Most of the foods that support emotional health have these two tastes. Why? Because they are the yang taste, about which we will learn more later. They can increase the body's quantity of yang energy and disperse energy up and out.

It is important not to consume too much of only one or two flavors. Usually we all enjoy the sweet, spicy and salty tastes, while the sour and bitter tastes are less desired. This can lead to an imbalance in the body. For instance, eating too much from the sweet food group can lead to weight gain and loss of muscle strength; an excess of salty food can lead to high blood pressure and an increase of water retention. That's why the World Health Organization encourages people to consume less than 6g of salt daily. Balancing the five flavors also has the benefit of expanding the variety of your diet.

When we try some flavors of food, like the bitter taste, we need to give our body three chances to determine whether it will accept or like this food or not. If you only try once, your body may not be able to tell.

The Chinese idiom *liang yao ku kou* (良药苦口) states that a food or herb with a bitter taste usually contains medicinal properties. This should make us realize that health benefits should be weighed along with taste preferences when making food choices. If there is some taste you really cannot take much of or do not like at all, when you understand its benefits, it may lessen your resistance and help you to make healthy choices.

4. Curing Health Problems

Whenever we face health problems, we should consider food first as a part of treatment. It is true that "you are what you eat." Your daily food intake molds your constitution and can influence well-being. Over the long-term, food consumption can even help in negating inherited disorders. The Chinese saying "illness comes from mouth" (*bing cong kou ru* 病 从 口 入) is still true for many diseases. Heart diseases, a fatty liver, high blood pressure, high cholesterol and weight gain very much have to do with our food intake. If we can reduce certain foods in the early stages of those illnesses, we can really take control of the condition and eventually return to a healthy state.

The same food can be used for different reasons. For example, in the southern part of China, people drink a lot of cooling tea during the hot summer months. However, people can benefit from cooling tea, even if the climate where they live is not as hot. For instance, they can drink cooling tea to cure hot ailments such as toothaches, bleeding gums, red eyes or flushed face. Therefore, it is important to note health factors when choosing foods.

Food therapy encourages us to think about food as our medicine when we face health issues. By reducing or increasing certain food items, we can manage many health conditions and get better much more quickly without the side effects often associated with pharmaceutical medicine.

5. Understanding the Role of Age, Sex and Constitution

It is important to choose only those foods that are compatible with our age, sex and constitution (more about constitution can be found in Chapter 2). For example, children, adults and seniors may not use the same ingredients or the same dosage to treat a symptom because their constitutions are different.

In the younger age group, people may tend to consume a great deal of fruits or vegetables as a main source of fiber. In China, people over the age of 80 do not consume much fruit during the winter months. Their source of fiber will be more from the root vegetables, like potatoes, sweet potatoes and taro, as this is better for their digestive system. This traces back to the famous Dr. Chen from the Song dynasty (960–1279), who encouraged elderly people to eat foods that are warm, cooked and soft, and to avoid foods that are glutinous, hardened, raw or cold. Because elderly people have weaker blood and essence, their digestive system function also decreases.

Health care in China also focuses on the special needs of different age groups. From the age of 24 to 35, people should focus on preventative measures. They should do all things in moderation (for example, food consumption or working hours), and keep a balanced emotional state. For this group it is best to choose more neutral ingredients.

From the age of 36 to 65, people should focus on preventing chronic and more serious illnesses, like high blood pressure, high cholesterol and high blood sugar. It is important to take notice of any hereditary diseases and take extra steps toward prevention. This age group should also be sure to consume foods that contain antioxidant properties.

At the age of 66 and above, health care should focus on harmonizing the organ systems (more on which can be found in Chapter 3). Special attention should be given to the digestive, circulatory, cardiovascular and metabolic systems. Regardless of whether or not they suffer from ailments, it is vital to keep our spleen and kidney systems healthy, as they are the foundations of our acquired constitution and congenital inheritance, respectively. The harmonization of the spleen and kidney systems helps in obtaining a high quality of life during later years.

Although the above rules apply generally, because women and men have different body constitutions, their health care can also be different. Since women have changes such as menstruation, pregnancy and post-partum in their life, they often need special foods to provide balance. For instance, Chinese angelica is only used for women. As for men, they have prostate glands and different reproductive structures than women, and they produce sperm and have regular ejaculation. Chinese chive seed is used mostly for men in regulating these functions.

In the following chapter, we provide tools for assessing your body constitution. As noted earlier, the constitution is a major concept in TCM, and it must be taken into consideration when selecting foods. Two women in same age group can have completely different food therapies because their constitutions are opposite. If Woman A has a hot constitution, she needs cool and cold foods to balance her body, while Woman B, with a cold constitution, needs to harmonize with warm and hot foods.

The following assessments will help you discover whether your constitution is balanced, cold or hot, damp or dry, weak or overly strong, or perhaps even a combination. Once you know your constitution, it will help you to choose, with this book as a guide, the correct ingredients to achieve a balance of yin and yang. For instance, if you have a dry constitution, select black sesame and wolfberries as cooling and neutral nourishment. However, you must be careful of not using too much or for too long, which might make your constitution overly damp.

Another approach to choosing food is to do so according to the organs and related meridians. If you have a dry constitution, the reason could be dryness in the lung or kidney. For dryness in the kidney, you would again use wolfberries and black sesame; however for dryness in the lung, lily bulbs or almond nut are recommended. To maximize the benefits, these ingredients should be used for at least one month.

Food therapy is based on the generalized constitution

combined with individual needs. Once you have achieved the right balance, you can once again enjoy a broad diet. Let's look now at how you can better understand your own body.

Chapter Two

Knowing Your Constitution

B ody constitution comprises our physical state, including the function of our internal systems and metabolism, together with our mental and spiritual states. As we pass through life, everyone's body constitution experiences periods of relative balance and imbalance, for example, passing from hot to cold or dry to damp. Imbalance of our body constitution could mark a transitional stage, when we are shifting away from health towards disorder, while not yet having a disease. Therefore, maintaining balance of body constitution can prevent or lessen disease and promote recovery from sickness.

Traditional Chinese medicine strives to balance the body's constitution, mitigate shocks from the outside environment, and dissolve toxic substances within our body.

1. Where Do Constitutions Come from?

Before we talk about using TCM methods for classifying different constitutions, we first need to understand more about the concept. What exactly is a constitution? Where does it come from? How can it be influenced?

The features of one's constitution can be detected in three areas: the physical build of the person, the body's internal functions, and the psychological state. It also depends on the stage of life the person is facing, such as puberty or menopause.

The constitution has two origins: congenital natural disposition and post-natal lifestyle (i.e. nature and nurture). Many factors influence the formation of the constitution: for instance, the parents' health, physically and mentally, at the time of conception, or the condition of the mother during pregnancy. These parts belong to the congenital natural disposition of one's constitution.

However, most of the influence comes from our own actions and lifestyle. We can examine these influences in six categories:

Diet
Regarding this most important influence, there are actually three

contributing categories. The first is basic healthy food that helps our body maintain itself on a daily basis. The second is food for pleasure, relaxing, socializing and as a response to satisfying certain emotional moods (in moderation, of course). The last is for the purpose of healing, reducing risks of illness, and maintaining and promoting good health.

Modern nutritional science is now, more than ever, researching this last category, as our bodies fight to stay in good health in a fast-paced and changing world. However, "functional food" or food as medicine, as we call this last category, has had 5,000 years of history in TCM.

Life Balance

Constitution is influenced by how one balances periods of work, stress and activity with those of calm, quiet and reflection. If we work long hours and do not have enough time to relax, or sometimes even not eat or sleep properly, our constitution will be out of balance. In TCM, there's a time for everything, and timing and schedule are crucial to maintaining a healthy constitution.

Our bodies move like a clock, with each organ channel having a two-hour period when there is a peak in its qi, the energy or life-process that flows in and around all of us. Qi flows clockwise through the twelve meridians over 24 hours, and shifts between yin and yang energies. We should eat three meals a day in order to refresh yang and yin energies (breakfast 7–9 a.m., lunch time 11 a.m.–1 p.m., and dinner 5–7 p.m.). It is best to start deep sleep between 11 p.m. and 1 a.m., and sleep well through 1 a.m. to 5 a.m., getting up and going to the toilet and moving the bowels in the period between 5 a.m.

and 7 a.m.

The times between breakfast and lunch, lunch and dinner, and dinner and sleep are the best times for physical and mental activities. As you can see, the best times to eat, sleep, work and think are all set out like clockwork in TCM!

Environment

Our surroundings affect our constitution, whether those influences are physical (such as weather, pollution or seasonal changes) or social/emotional (friends, co-workers and support systems). Natural environmental influences are not only external since they affect the water and food we put in our bodies. Therefore a healthy environment could protect your constitution.

Sexual Relationship and Conception

In a relationship, partners can affect each others' constitutions. A balance of sexual activity is needed to maintain harmony in a relationship; too little or too much can influence the balance of the body.

Similarly, when women do not conceive, they also show signs of disharmony in the body because pregnancy is a natural cycle in a woman's lifetime. The absence of pregnancy can cause the under-development of some meridian systems. Even women who decide not to breastfeed can show signs of blockage in the liver and stomach meridians due to the inability to access certain meridians connected to the action of releasing milk from the body. Frequent pregnancy is also a disharmonizing situation for some women with weaker constitutions.

Illness

Disease and other harmful conditions can change one's constitution. During the period when people fall ill, their body qi, blood, and yin and yang of their viscera are disturbed because of the harmful pathogenic factors. Normally, when one recovers, these changes also mend gradually, and should not alter the overall constitution.

However, certain special circumstances, such as a serious

and long-term illness, can cause lasting damage. If the body is not sufficiently restored and balanced after illness, the body constitution becomes weak. For example, if a patient experiences long-term chronic hemorrhages or overly heavy menstruation, it can easily cause an excessive qi and blood deficiency, forming a weak constitution.

Age and Gender

The constitution of infants features puerile yin-yang and tender organ systems, especially the digestive and respiratory systems. If an infant has a weak constitution, diligent care can gradually bring about a shift to a vigorous and healthy constitution in adolescence. On the contrary, even if the original constitution is good, poor nutrition and habits in childhood can cause the constitution to become increasingly weak in adolescence.

Similarly, constitution is subject to changes during other periods of life. During retirement years, kidney essence is decreased and yin-yang balance levels are downcast, resulting in a tendency more toward fear, fatigue and lonely feelings, which shows a weakening of the constitution. The body functions, as well as the structure of each system, progressively recede during this phase.

Menopause marks a period of transition from adulthood into old age. It involves both women and men, but in women is more obvious. It has a different effect on each individual based on the degree of balance in the constitution.

The properties of yin and yang are different; similarly, the properties of the male and female body are different. Males build up more yang, showing tall, strong and stable body characteristics. Their constitutions are more hot and strong. Females build up more yin, so that their outward appearance is slender, soft and flexible. Their constitutions are more cold and weak. Therefore men and women have many differences in their physiological functions, and their psychological state and coping abilities are different as well. This is determined by gender itself.

2. Assessing Your Body Constitution

To achieve balance and longevity, it is paramount to understand one's constitution, and the factors that influence it. The basis of TCM is rooted in this understanding, which is then used to create treatment plans that will bring one's health to an optimal level. These highly-individualized remedies include changing lifestyle habits and diet, and taking supplements.

Our body has its own internal program, quite like a climate control system in a home. Such a system can automatically adjust according to season, cooling a home in the summer while heating it in winter, or controlling dampness in the spring and adding moisture to the dry autumn air. These systems are carefully balanced. They need power to run, and wires and pipelines to make a complete system.

Although we may not realize it, our bodies are also automatically regulating our metabolism to adapt to seasonal changes. For example, if our bodies cannot properly warm up in the winter, we will feel cold, which may lead to a lack of energy. We need to assist and fine-tune our body's natural regulation system. One of the best and most natural ways to repair our system and maintain equilibrium is through the use of proper foods and herbs.

Like the one in our home, the "control system" of our body also relies on power and a network of connections. The body's power comes through our blood and qi. The blood vessels serve as a sort of visible power wire, while the meridians, which connect major organ systems, are invisible.

Recently, there has been a resurgence of an ancient and fundamental principle of traditional Chinese medicine: the classification of different constitutions. Modern TCM focuses on determining constitution based on the state of one's blood and qi. A person must understand his or her own constitution in order to take the right steps to find good health. The assessments below will help you learn more about your own constitution in order to choose foods and herbs specifically suited to your individual needs.

Questions Relating to Temperature:
Neutral, Cold, Hot or Mixed Constitution

1) Are you sensitive to the cold or heat?
   - ☐ normal (1)
   - ☐ sensitive to cold (2)
   - ☐ sensitive to heat (3)
2) What do you prefer to drink?
   - ☐ depends on season (1)
   - ☐ warm/hot drinks (2)
   - ☐ cold drinks (3)
3) Do you sweat a lot?
   - ☐ normal (1)
   - ☐ less than average (2)
   - ☐ more than average (3)
4) How do you classify your thirst?
   - ☐ normal (1)
   - ☐ not often thirsty (2)
   - ☐ often thirsty (3)
5) How is your complexion?
   - ☐ shining and rosy (1)
   - ☐ pale and puffy (2)
   - ☐ flushed (3)
6) How is your tongue coating when you get up in the morning?
   - ☐ thin white fur (1)
   - ☐ thick white fur (2)
   - ☐ thick yellow fur (3)
7) What is your pulse (beats per minute)?
   - ☐ from 60 to 80 (1)
   - ☐ less than 60 (2)
   - ☐ over 80 (3)
8) Do you like tea or coffee?
   - ☐ up to two cups of coffee or tea every day (1)
   - ☐ three or more cups of tea every day (2)
   - ☐ three or more cups of coffee every day (3)
9) What kind of food do you prefer?
   - ☐ depends on season (1)

☐ a light taste or raw food (2)
☐ spicy or strongly flavored (3)

Assessment:
Neutral: 6 or more responses of (1)
Cold: 6 or more of (2)
Hot: 6 of more of (3)
Mixed: if fewer than 6 of any one response

Cold or hot

Questions Relating to Humidity:
Neutral, Damp, Dry or Mixed Constitution

1) What is your tongue like?
  ☐ normal size with a thin white coating (1)
  ☐ large with a thick or wet coating (2)
  ☐ small with a thin or dry coating (3)
2) What kind of taste do you usually have in your mouth?
  ☐ normal (1)
  ☐ sticky and sweet (2)
  ☐ dry (3)
3) What is your skin condition?
  ☐ normal or mixed (1)
  ☐ oily (2)
  ☐ dry or cracking (3)
4) How would you characterize your excretion? (Discharge from eyes, ears and skin; for women, includes monthly period)
  ☐ comfortable amount (1)
  ☐ quite a lot (2)
  ☐ scant or absent (3)
5) Do you smoke or drink alcohol?
  ☐ occasionally (1)
  ☐ frequently (2)
  ☐ refrain from both (3)
6) What is your tolerance for dairy products?
  ☐ average (1)

☐ less than average (2)
☐ more than average (3)

7) How do you feel in general?
    ☐ happy and relaxed (1)
    ☐ heavy, sleepy; fullness of chest and stomach (2)
    ☐ irritable, anxious; dry lips and throat (3)

8) How would you characterize your bowel movements and urine output?
    ☐ normal (1)
    ☐ loose stool or turbid urine (2)
    ☐ dry stool, constipation or scanty urine (3)

9) How would you describe your build?
    ☐ average (1)
    ☐ heavy build (2)
    ☐ slim (3)

Assessment:
Neutral: 6 or more responses of (1)
Damp: 6 or more of (2)
Dry: 6 or more of (3)
Mixed: if fewer than 6 of any one response

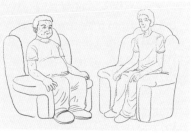

Damp or dry

Questions Regarding Your Response to Adversity:
Neutral, Weak, Overly Strong or Mixed Constitution

1) Do you feel energetic?
    ☐ average (1)
    ☐ more than average (2)
    ☐ less than average (3)

2) What is your tongue like when you get up in the morning?
    ☐ pink body and thin fur (1)
    ☐ dark or purple body and thick fur (2)
    ☐ pale or deeper red body and no fur (3)

3) What kind of food you prefer?
    ☐ mixed, with more vegetables and less meat (1)

☐ mostly meat (2)

☐ vegetarian (3)

4) How often is your elimination?

☐ normal (1)

☐ infrequent (2)

☐ too frequent (3)

5) How often do you get a cold every year?

☐ once or a few times (1)

☐ never (2)

☐ often (3)

6) How often do you get excited?

☐ normal (1)

☐ frequently (2)

☐ seldom (3)

7) How do your muscles feel?

☐ normal (1)

☐ tight and sore (2)

☐ soft and weak (3)

8) How quickly do you feel shortness of breath when hiking?

☐ 15 minutes to half an hour (1)

☐ more than half an hour (2)

☐ after a few minutes (3)

9) How does your head often feel?

☐ normal (1)

☐ pressure or sharp headache (2)

☐ lightheaded or dizziness (3)

Assessment:
Neutral: 6 or more responses of (1)
Weak: 6 or more of (3)
Overly Strong: 6 or more of (2)
Mixed: if fewer than 6 of any one response

Weak or overly strong

In completing the above self-assessment, we encounter some pairs of concepts: cold or hot, damp or dry, weak or overly strong. All these feelings, when within a certain range, are normal for us to feel. We should feel cold in winter and hot in summer. However, if we always feel cold, even in spring, or feel cold too often, then we should seek the underlying reason and try to remedy it.

The approach toward damp and dry is similar; both are necessary and normal within boundaries. Dampness nourishes our inside and moistens the surface of skin while dryness limits the growth of mold. However, too much damp makes skin oily and develop acne. In turn, too much dryness brings wrinkles and cracking. Therefore we should stay in neutral as long as we can.

Now that you have assessed your constitution, we can use that information in choosing the right foods and herbs to help you achieve and maintain balance.

Let's take damp, dry and neutral constitutions as an example. If you have a result of a neutral type, it means you are quite balanced. In order to keep this state, it is best to eat a broad range of foods and be sure to drink water according to the climate and your level of perspiration. However, if you have a damp constitution, this means there is too much humidity inside of you. You need to add specific foods to your diet (such as pearl barley, red beans, corn or winter squash) to reduce dampness and bring yourself back to balance. A dry type, on the other hand, would have different requirements for a healthy diet. In this case, foods such as lily bulb, Chinese wolfberry, honey or lemon can nourish and moisten the body. Chapter Four will tell you more about the specific foods and herbs best suited to your constitution.

Chapter Three

Choosing the Right Foods and Herbs for a Balanced Constitution

The basis of the "functional food" approach is to match the appropriate foods and herbs to the corresponding body constitutions. As we have seen in the previous chapter, the body constitution can be overly strong or weak, hot or cold, dry or damp, or mixed. Foods and herbs also have inherent properties; they have different temperatures and tastes, and they enter different channels of the body. The proper use of food can correct the body's extremes, bringing a property that is out of proportion back into balance. It can, so to speak, yin our yang, yang our yin, strengthen our weakness, calm our hyperactivity, cool our heat, warm our cold, moisten our dryness and dispel our dampness to achieve optimal health.

Now before we look at the features of food and their application, we must understand some basic concepts underlying TCM theory: Yin and Yang, the Five Elements, and the Meridians and Organ Systems.

1. Yin-Yang Theory

Mark, a 26-year-old, often felt hot and irritable, perspired a lot no matter the time of day or season, and had trouble adapting to hot weather. He enjoyed cold or iced drinks and couldn't tolerate spicy food. After a TCM consultation, he began to drink more mint and lemon tea, and to reduce his coffee intake. Gradually, his perspiring stopped. He is now beginning to enjoy warm weather and to feel less distracted and irritable.

What does this example tell us about yin and yang, an ancient philosophical concept that is so central to TCM? Yin and yang are two fundamental principles or forces in the universe, ever opposing and supplementing each other. All things and phenomena in the

Yin and yang

natural world contain two opposite components, for example, heaven/earth or heat/cold. In TCM, yin and yang properties can be assigned to one's constitution as well as the food and herbs that one consumes.

A yang constitution includes hot, dry and overly strong properties of different body systems, while yin constitutions demonstrate cold, damp and weak properties. Yin foods, such as watermelon and mung bean, can bring nourishment and moisture internally as well as to the skin and orifices. They can reduce heat and calm the mind. Yang foods, such as walnut and cinnamon, can warm and energize the body, dry dampness and stimulate metabolism. Neutral foods, such as mushrooms, provide nutrition while not influencing body temperature.

TCM uses food to balance constitutions. For example, if a person's constitution has too much yang, it can be neutralized by yin food. In the example with the patient Mark above, the mint and lemon, which are yin foods, balanced his yang symptoms.

Origin and Principles of Yin and Yang

We should now step back a moment and explore the basic concept of yin and yang more thoroughly. In the beginning, yin and yang described a place's location in relation to the sun. A place exposed to the sun is yang, and a place without exposure is yin. The southern side of a mountain, for example, is yang, while its northern side is yin. Thus the ancient Chinese people, in the course of their everyday life and work, came to understand that all aspects of the natural world could be seen as having a dual aspect, for example, day and night, brightness and dimness, movement and stillness, upward and downward.

The terms yin and yang were applied to express these dual and opposite qualities. Chapter Five of the ancient TCM classic book of *Plain Questions* states that "water and fire are symbols of yin and yang," so we can remember the features of yin and yang by comparing them with water and fire, or things that embody similar opposites, such as the sun and moon. In China, this method of describing people is commonplace; for example, when a boy is open-minded, vigorous and optimistic, he is called a "sunny boy."

The content of the theory of yin and yang can be described briefly as follows: opposition, interdependence, relative waxing and waning, and transformation.

Opposition and Interdependence of Yin and Yang

By the opposition of yin and yang, we mean that all things and phenomena in the natural world contain two opposite components: heaven and earth, outside and inside, movement and stability, etc. In the theory of yin and yang, heaven is considered yang, while earth is yin; outside is yang, while inside is yin; movement is yang, while stability is yin.

Yin and yang not only oppose but also contain each other. Without the other, neither can exist. For instance, without outside, there would be no inside, and vice versa. This relationship of coexistence is known as interdependence. TCM holds that "functional movement" belongs to yang, "nourishing substance" to yin, and that the one cannot exist without the other.

The Waxing and Waning of Yin and Yang and the Transformation between Yin and Yang

Yin and yang are not stagnant but exist in a dynamic state—while yin wanes, yang waxes, and vice versa. This dynamic change of succeeding each other is known as the waxing and waning of yin and yang. Take the seasonal climatic variation in the natural world for example. The weather gets warm when winter gives way to spring, and becomes hot when spring gives way to summer, during which time yin wanes while yang waxes. However, it gets cool when autumn replaces summer, and cold when winter replaces autumn, during which time yang wanes but yin waxes.

By "transformation," we mean that yin and yang will transform into one another under certain conditions. For instance, in the course of suffering from a disease, a patient may run a high fever, have a red complexion, feel irritable and restless, and have a rapid and strong pulse—indicating strong yang. But all of a sudden, he may show yin characteristics, feeling listless, with a low temperature, pale face and weak pulse. This is an example of transformation from yang to yin.

Uses of Yin-Yang Theory in TCM

Yin-yang theory has had an integral impact on the science of TCM, and its basic principles have played an important role in the formation and development of TCM's own theoretical system. It is used to explain the tissues and structures, physiology functions and pathology changes of the human body, and to direct clinical diagnosis and treatment. It also forms a basis for the clinical application of Chinese food and medicinal herbs. In doing so, one can achieve the aim of curing diseases.

When a patient visits a TCM clinic, the doctor will seek to understand the patient's symptoms according to yin-yang theory. For example, when categorizing the characteristics of the face and tongue, as well as bodily excretions, the colors red, yellow and green belong to yang, while white and gray belong to yin. A diagnosis is established on the basis of the predominance or weakness of yin and yang. This guides treatment, as foods and herbs are selected according to their property of yin or yang. A basic summary of this process is in the table below.

	Yin	Yang
Symptoms	Cold limbs, pale face, pale tongue with a white coating, affinity for hot drinks	Burning or heat in the body, red face, red tongue with yellow coating, affinity for cold or iced drinks
TCM diagnosis	Yin pattern	Yang pattern
Remedy	Consume food and herbs with yang characteristics	Consume food and herbs with yin characteristics

Yang and Yin: The Temperature of Foods and Herbs

Let's examine what is meant by yang and yin foods and herbs. Yang means the "temperature" of the food is warm or hot; this is an inherent property and not necessarily dependant on the surface temperature of the food. The "taste," a concept we will learn more about in the section below on the Five Elements, can be pungent, sweet or bland.

Yang foods are more likely to be seasonal foods found in the winter. Cooking or preparation methods include stir-frying, stewing, baking, deep-frying, roasting, grilling or barbecue. These foods and herbs make our body energy rise and come to the surface.

Yin means the temperature of the food is cool or cold, and the taste is sour, bitter or salty. These foods are most plentifully found in the summer, and are often eaten raw or steamed. Yin foods restrain our body's energy or cause it to descend.

There are also a lot of foods that have very mild yin or yang qualities, and therefore belong to "neutral" food. Examples include rice, corn, kale and carrots. Even if you do not have detailed knowledge about the yin and yang of food, if you consume a broad range of foods, you can quite naturally get a balance of yin and yang.

2. The Five Elements

In Chinese, the Five Elements are called Wu Xing—Wu means five and Xing means movement and change. The Five Elements—wood, fire, earth, metal and water—have their own specific properties, but they also play interactive functions of generation and restriction. For example, earth generates metal but restricts water, while earth, in turn, is restricted by wood. This means that the relationship between the elements is one of constant motion and change.

Together, the concepts of yin-yang and the Five Elements form the basis of traditional Chinese medical theory. They help explain the functions and relationships of different parts of the body, and guide clinical diagnosis and treatment.

The therapeutic use of food in TCM is partly based on the Five Element model, as each food or herb has a certain "color" and "taste" related to one of the elements. In determining a food's "color," the inside color is considered more than the skin color. The "taste" of a food or herb is not always related to its flavor. For instance, while the taste of broccoli is classified as "bitter" and millet as "salty," it relates more to an intrinsic quality rather than its actual flavor, although in most cases the two will coincide.

Before exploring more about taste and flavor, we will first look at how Five Elements theory is used to classify things in nature, including the human body.

Classification

Based on Five Elements theory, TCM has made a comprehensive study of all things in nature and attributed them respectively to one of the Five Elements in accordance with their different properties, functions and forms. This approach to understanding the physiology and pathology of the human body makes a strong correlation between humans and their natural surroundings. The tables below demonstrate how things are classified according to Five Elements theory (more about *zang* and *fu* organs can be found in the following section about meridians).

Five Elements and the Human Body					
Element	*Zang*-Organ	*Fu*-Organ	Sense Organ	Tissue	Emotion
Wood	Liver	Gall bladder	Eye	Tendons	Anger
Fire	Heart	Small Intestine	Tongue	Vessels	Joy
Earth	Spleen	Stomach	Mouth	Muscles	Thinking
Metal	Lung	Large Intestine	Nose	Skin and Body Hair	Worry
Water	Kidney	Urinary Bladder	Ear and lower orifices	Bone	Fear

Five Elements and Nature						
Element	Season	Environmental Factor	Growth & Development	Color	Taste	Orientation
Wood	Spring	Wind	Germination	Blue (green)	Sour	East
Fire	Summer	Heat	Growth	Red	Bitter	South
Earth	Last 18 days of each season, Rainy Season	Dampness	Transformation	Yellow	Sweet	Middle
Metal	Autumn	Dryness	Reaping	White	Pungent (spicy)	West
Water	Winter	Cold	Storing	Black	Salty	North

Applying the Five Elements in Food Therapy—Color

The color and taste of foods indicate an essential quality in that food, describing a potential that is liberated by the alchemy of cooking and digestion. As seen in the table above, Five Elements theory holds that different colors of foods or herbs correspond with different organ systems and seasons. Each color and flavor arises from one elemental power and is said to enter a particular meridian and organ.

Green: Corresponds with the liver system. Green foods are best for spring. They can regulate liver qi, helping the liver to dispel toxins from the body. Too much alcohol and rich protein can harm the liver. There is a high relapse rate for liver ailments in spring, especially chronic ones. Green foods are usually rich in fiber, vitamins and chlorophyll, which help in cleansing toxins.

Red: Corresponds with the heart system. Red foods are best for summer. They help nourish blood, improve circulation, and reinforce yang (warm) energy. They are usually recommended for people with anemia, palpitations, cold limbs, paleness and weakness.

Yellow: Corresponds with the spleen system (digestive system), assists digestion and helps reinforce spleen energy. Yellow foods are suitable year-round, but are particularly good for the rainy season. Yellow foods, like soybeans and pumpkins, are usually rich in vitamins A and D. Vitamin A can protect the lining in the digestive and respiratory systems, which helps prevent stomach inflation and ulcers. Vitamin D promotes the absorption of calcium and phosphorus, thus strengthening bones.

White: Corresponds with the lung system. White foods are best for autumn, providing one of the best remedies for the dryness of the season. Apart from relieving coughing, they can also help nourish skin and fight constipation through the promotion of body fluids. White foods such as milk, lily bulb and fish are also recommended by nutritionists as they are rich in protein yet relatively low in fat.

Black: Corresponds with the kidney system. Black foods are best for winter, a season when, according to TCM, one should store energy. The kidney system plays a role in this, and black foods promote and strengthen the kidney system. Otherwise, people with a poor kidney system will miss many of the benefits of the reinforcing foods eaten in winter. Research shows that most black foods are rich in inorganic salt and melanin. The inorganic salt can help promote fluid metabolism and dispel toxins, while melanin restricts nitrosamine, thus helping to prevent cancer.

Applying the Five Elements in Food Therapy—Taste

Five Elements theory also states that each of the tastes has certain effects on the body as described below.

Sour: This taste helps with digestive absorption, resisting fatty foods and preventing indigestion. It generates fluids and yin, and stops discharge, perspiration, chronic cough and diarrhea. It also has an astringent effect on emissions, including sperm and frequent urine. It helps our body consolidate essential substances, preventing them from escape. Sour foods can also bring disordered qi back to normal. Modern research shows sour flavors to be generally cleansing and detoxifying. However, we have to limit intake when ulcer or stones are present.

Bitter: This taste clears away heat, calms body and dries dampness. It can control abnormally ascending qi and purge any pathogenic fire effect. In certain combinations, it can also improve the body's yin. Bitter foods can be used to treat most cases of excess and acute damp-heat or heat-fire. These foods should be limited if a weakness of qi and blood is present.

Sweet: Serving to nourish, moisten, moderate and invigorate the body, sweet foods can also regulate qi, blood and function of the viscera. They strengthen deficiency syndrome and alleviate dryness. Sweet foods work in coordination with the spleen and stomach. They can help relieve pain and spasms, and reduce cough, ulcer and constipation. An excess of sweets should be avoided when suffering from damp, phlegm and water retention conditions.

Spicy (pungent): This taste disperses and promotes movement of qi and blood circulation. It stimulates digestion and helps break through blockage. It treats syndromes of the exterior, and expels stagnation of qi, blood and pathogens. Spicy foods must be used carefully as many people cannot tolerate them. Caution should also be taken when suffering from an acute disease with heat type of condition.

Salty: These foods can promote moisture and have a softening effect. In particular, these foods regulate the moisture balance flow downwards in the body. They also move qi downward, increase urine and bowel movements, and are used to treat constipation and swelling. They promote the action of the kidney system, allowing beneficial foods to be fully absorbed and functional, and improving concentration. Salty foods soften nodes and masses, and disperse accumulations in hardening muscles and glands.

Bland: This taste promotes urination and treats edema.

Bringing Balance to Your Diet

Effectiveness of a food may be compromised by other underlying conditions. It should also be noted that small and moderate amounts of a food are beneficial while excess is harmful. For example, over dosage of the sour taste can upset the liver, so it should be used sparingly if a person suffers from chronic pain. Bitter taste affects the bones, so an excess of it should be avoided by those with bone diseases. Sweet foods work on the muscles, and taking too much can cause muscle weakness. Since the pungent taste scatters qi, it should be avoided in cases of qi weakness. Finally, the salty taste can dry the blood, and it should be avoided by those with blood deficiency.

The fundamental TCM book *Huangdi Neijing*, also known as the *Yellow Emperor's Inner Cannon*, states that when we eat, we should "mediate the five flavors carefully." This concept may not be in our mind, ordinarily, as we walk around a supermarket or look into our refrigerators. However, using this philosophy as a basic guide when choosing foods helps to balance our diet and eat food that is functional for our own body.

3. Meridians and Organ Systems

The view of Chinese medicine is that the body-mind network is an integrated whole. The conception of the Meridians and Organ Systems reflects this view, representing a landscape of functional relationships that provide total integration of bodily functions, emotions, mental activities, tissues, sense organs and environmental influences.

Classification

The holistic approach is based on the five *zang* organs. These are defined much more broadly than in Western medicine, including not only the organ but its entire functional system, linked via meridians. The meridians are communication lines between all parts of the body—pathways that carry qi, blood and body fluids.

Heart system: heart—small intestine—blood vessels—tongue

The heart is in control of the body's physical and psychological functions. It not only governs the blood and circulation, but it is also the storehouse of the spirit. The heart system opens onto the tongue. In Western medicine, it would be roughly equivalent to the circulatory and cranial nervous systems.

Liver system: liver—gall bladder—tendons—eyes

The liver stores blood, controls the tendons, and governs the conducting, dispersion and smooth flow of qi. This regulates both emotional health and digestive function. The system opens into the eyes. Its functions relate to part of the Western circulatory, peripheral nervous and digestive systems.

Spleen system: spleen—stomach—muscles—mouth

The spleen is the source of acquired constitution, meaning all the factors that develop post-natally. Directing transformation and transportation, it governs blood flow within the vessels. This system controls the muscles and limbs, and opens into the pharynx and mouth. It is related to digestion, water metabolism and the hemopoietic system in Western medicine.

Lung system: lung—large intestine—skin and body hair—nose

The lung receives messages from the heart and administers these signals throughout the body, especially producing and regulating the body's qi. It controls the circulation and regulates the body's metabolism of fluid. The lung controls the skin, and the system opens into the larynx and nose. The approximate Western equivalent is the respiratory system and processes involved in fluid regulation.

Kidney system: kidney—urinary bladder—bone—ears and lower orifices

The kidney is responsible for the body's overall constitution, and is the congenital base of life. It is a storage facility for good essence, and it governs the growth and development of the body as well as the reproductive systems. It governs water metabolism and the reception and transformation of qi. The kidney system controls the bones, producing marrow, and opens into the ears and two lower orifices. It can be seen as equivalent to the urogential and endocrine system, as well as part of the nervous system.

The meridians have a close relationship with the organ systems. They are the passages by which the *zang*, or major organs (for example, the heart) and *fu*, or secondary organs (for example, the small intestine) connect with one another.

The relationships between the liver, heart, spleen, lung and kidney show these connections. In the meridian system, the liver meridian and the gallbladder meridian run through the heart; the liver meridian runs on both sides of the stomach, which is part of the spleen system; the kidney meridian ascends and runs through the liver; the liver meridian ascends to the lung; and so on. By means of these interconnecting meridians, the five systems maintain relative balance and coordination.

Application in Food Therapy—Channels of Entry

Over its long history, Chinese medicine has come to realize that different foods enter specific meridian pathways, directing their effect towards particular organs. This information directs the therapeutic use of the food. When we know which meridian and/ or organ a food will target, this is useful in treating a disorder of that particular meridian or organ. For instance, onion enters the lung meridian and lung, while the lychee targets the liver meridian and liver. Peppers affect the stomach meridian and stomach; sunflower seeds, the spleen meridian and spleen; kidney beans, naturally, the kidney meridian and kidney; and coffee, the heart and its meridian.

Another approach to choosing food is to do so according to the organs and related meridians. If you have a dry constitution, the reason could be dryness in the lung or the kidney. As noted earlier, for dryness in the kidney, you can choose wolfberries and black sesame, while for dryness in the lung, lily bulbs or almond nut are best. If you have a tendency to feel cold in your stomach area, you should add ginger tea to your diet. You can also add ginger and spring onion to food. To maximize the benefits, use these ingredients for at least one month.

4. Three Major Beliefs about Food in Chinese Medicine

1) **Food is the cornerstone of life.** It nourishes, provides vitamins and minerals, promotes growth, and enhances longevity; it is life-sustaining. Functional food can also help to prevent or treat certain illnesses.

2) **Some foods can be harmful or cause illness.** In some people or under certain conditions, foods can cause acute or immediate reactions and problems. Examples include allergies, food poisoning, symptoms related to lactose intolerance, etc. Timing and amount of food consumption can also negatively impact the digestive system, such as prolonged hunger or long periods between meals, or eating and drinking too much at one meal. Over-eating one type of food also has a negative effect. An example is a patient who exercised regularly and ate healthy in every way, including a heavily vegetable-based diet, except that she ate dark chocolate every day and was later diagnosed with high cholesterol.

Another way that food can harm is when people eat foods that don't agree with their body. As we know, TCM believes that individual bodies may be more inclined to "hot" or "cold" constitutions. Those who are on the hot side may experience more constipation, heartburn or mouth ulcers. If this is the case, they should avoid foods that raise the heat in the body, such as spicy foods, coffee or hot soups. By contrast, people who are in the cold spectrum may have an upset stomach from drinking too many cold drinks, eating ice cream, and so on, and therefore should avoid raw foods or other cold foods that make them feel ill, even if they enjoy the flavor.

To avoid excess in eating certain types of foods, you should be mindful of your flavor preference or aversion. Continually eating from only one flavor group can negatively impact various organs. For example, eating only spicy foods can make you sweat too much and reduce water content in the body, making the lungs dry out. Likewise, too much salt can negatively impact the kidneys as they struggle to filter properly. People who eat many sweet things, such as cookies or anything with added sugar, will often face problems with their pancreas from over stimulation and too much insulin production.

3) Undigested food becoming stagnant in the digestive tract can lead to chronic ailments. This may happen if food is not digested thoroughly the first time, if it is not passed in a timely manner, or if particles become stuck in the intestines. Signs that food has accumulated in the digestive tract may include poor appetite, belching or gas with a distinct smell, bloating or diarrhea, and in severe cases, painful heartburn with a bitter taste in the throat and mouth. When not resolved, gastritis, irritable bowel syndrome (IBS), pancreatitis and gallstones are likely to occur; polyps can also develop in the colon, leading to colon cancer.

Foods and herbs have specific therapeutic actions beyond their temperature, color and taste, or the meridians traveled. A food may either tonify/strengthen a particular substance or function (qi, blood, yin and yang) or it may reduce or regulate the influence of a pathological condition (qi or blood stagnation, dampness, heat or cold). Lychee, for example, reduces cold and regulates blood circulation to treat pigmentation on the face. Kidney bean tonifies yang.

Therefore, we need to put all the qualities of food together to fully understand its therapeutic effect. For example, people with a cold constitution can choose red wine or pomegranate, but they need to understand first that red wine enters all meridians, while pomegranate enters the lung, kidney and large intestine meridian. Similarly, those with hot constitutions might choose green tea, which enters the heart, stomach and kidney meridians. Another choice is the blueberry, which enters the lung, spleen and stomach meridians. Body constitution, food temperature, taste and the meridians it travels must be considered to choose the food perfect for you.

This tailor-made knowledge helps in judging individual needs when we choose functional food, herbs and supplements. There are so many choices out there, and decisions can often be made on superficial terms, influenced by packaging or advertising. However, if you understand the basics of Chinese medicine, your choices will be wiser, allowing foods to work holistically to help you get and stay healthy.

Chapter Four

Functional Foods and Herbs from A-Z

In this chapter, we will explore the details of each functional food and herb, learning how to use them therapeutically following the principles of TCM. The common English, Chinese and Latin names are used to ensure you get the correct foods. Information about the native geographical location (focusing on China) will help you select those grown at their point of origin. If you cannot get foods from their native location, use similar foods from the same family.

The healthy benefits discussed here come from traditional Chinese medicine food therapy supplemented by the application of new therapeutic techniques developed through modern research, including extensive pharmacological investigations.

The "How to eat" section of each entry incorporates both Chinese and Western ways of eating, although the majority are Chinese methods of preparation. The "Decoction" preparation method listed for many of the foods and herbs uses boiling to extract and concentrate dissolved chemicals or herbal or plant material. The "Contraindication" section relies on the clinical experience accumulated during generations of practice by TCM doctors. Before attempting to prepare any of these remedies, you may want to read the Appendices "Getting Ready" and "Cooking Techniques" so that you are efficient and accurate.

All foods and herbs, including supplements, come from plants that have their own individual characteristics: temperatures, flavors, reactions to meridians, and therapeutic functions. It is therefore vital to understand your constitution in order to determine which plants will work for you. So please be sure to take the self-assessment in Chapter Two before using the information that follows here.

The foods and herbs discussed in this section can be divided into ten basic groups, each with its own function:

1) Cool the body
2) Warm the body
3) Improve blood circulation
4) Eliminate dampness and water retention
5) Stimulate the movement of qi
6) Nourish and hydrate the body
7) Tonify (increase/strengthen) qi and yang energy
8) Detoxify the body
9) Calm the mind and regulate emotions
10) Aid digestion

Almond (Apricot Kernel) 甜杏仁

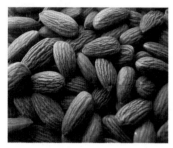

Scientific name and origin: Almonds are seeds of Rosaceae, with the Latin name of *Armeniaca vulgaris* Lam. Within China, almonds are primarily grown in Jiangsu, Shandong, Anhui and Shaanxi provinces.

Properties and taste: Neutral; sweet

Channels of entry: Lung and large intestine

Composition and pharmacology: Almonds are a good source of calcium, which can help in the prevention of osteoporosis. Almonds may help reduce the risk of colon cancer. The polyphenols in almonds help prevent the oxidation of LDL cholesterol, while the high content of healthy monounsaturated fat is also effective in reducing cholesterol. The potassium in almonds provides protection against high blood pressure and atherosclerosis. Almonds appear to reduce post-meal elevation in blood sugar levels, which is helpful for diabetics.

Culinary usage and medical applications:

1. Moisturizing the lung, relieving asthma: Almond dispels phlegm, relieves asthma, nourishes the lungs and causes counter-rising qi to come down. Almond treats chronic and weak coughs, and prevents dry throat. Eating 6–9g can remove pressure from the chest area.

2. Moisturizing the large intestine, eliminating constipation: It helps dry stool and eases the motion of the colon.

How to eat?

1. Raw or roasted: Sweet almond can be eaten in this way, generally 6–9g a day.

2. Powder: Mix with cereal and oatmeal.

3. Decoction: With gingko nut to treat productive cough and asthma.

Contraindication:

Some people cannot tolerate almonds well; it is best to not eat more than 200g per day.

Almonds are not to be used to treat acute flu or cough.

Avoid eating almonds if you have loose stools.

Aloe Vera and Aloe Vera Granule
芦荟 芦荟粉

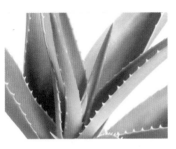

Scientific name and origin: Aloe is derived from *Aloe vera* (L.) Burm. f. The family name is the Aloaceae. The aloe vera granule is the concentrated liquid from the succulent stem aloe. *A. vera* is grown in northern Africa, South and North American, and the West Indies.

Properties and taste: Cold; bitter

Channels of entry: Liver, stomach and large intestine

Composition and pharmacology: Aloe contains free amino acids, 21 kinds of organic acid, and vitamins, bradykinin, anthraquinones class, phenols and nucleoside, etc. Aloe is known to strengthen the immune system when taken internally and promote faster wound healing when applied externally. Aloe prevents constipation and can induce diarrhea. It also protects the liver and seems to have an anti-bacterial, anti-inflammatory and anti-tumor effects. Many of the aloe juice products on the North American market are filtered to remove the anthraquinones. Because of this, they often do not cause diarrhea. The primary portion of the plant that causes diarrhea is the latex exudates. Most of the "granules" also lack the anthraquinones.

Culinary usage and medical applications:

1. Relieving constipation by purgation: "Heat" in the digestive tract may be indicated by poor colon function, hunger followed quickly by feeling full, facial acne and/or bad breath throughout the day. Its primary treatment is the application of

aloe. After passing a stool, cease use of aloe.

2. Cooling liver heat: Aloe can cool liver heat as evidenced by red face and eyes, constipation, seething or silent anger, scant dark yellow urine, or a sense of fullness in the upper abdominal region.

3. Destroying parasites: Eat fresh aloe with mume fruit juice (also known as Chinese plum, scientific name *Prunus mume*), or aloe granules combined with mume fruit tea. This is to treat children suffering from abdominal pain with white patches on face and nails caused by roundworm.

4. External use: Aloe, usually as a gel, can be used directly on the skin for acne, sunburn, athlete's foot and to stop bleeding. Alternately, mix dried aloe powder or freshly juiced aloe (up to 5–7% concentration) with other acne-reducing face cream and apply directly on the affected area; don't apply to the whole face. It can also help urticaria and psoriasis due to heat.

How to eat?
Fresh

1. Raw or juice: Eat fresh or juiced to aid digestion, or mixed with honey and used instead of jam on toast. Fresh juice is recommended for people with one of more of the following symptoms: painful constipation, fullness, distention, irritability or scant dark urine. Be careful not to drink too much, particularly too much fresh extract, as it could lead to diarrhea, irritation of the stomach lining, or in excess doses, miscarriage.

2. Steeped into tea: Recurring urinary tract infections (UTI) can be treated with aloe. Using fresh cut aloe, cook first for 5 minutes and then steep into tea. Or you can drink pure fresh aloe juice or extract, up to 8ml per day.

3. Aloe wine: Put fresh cut aloe into a bowl or jar, add Chinese distilled liquor at the ratio of 1.5:1 (aloe: wine). Store in a cool, dark area for 4 weeks before drinking.

Dried

1. Tea: If only dried aloe is available, it can be made into tea, or you can mix dried aloe into other drinks.

2. Powder: Mix with other herbs to make pills or put powder

into a capsule then take 1–2 capsules a day for constipation or fat in blood.

Contraindication:

Pregnant women must not take aloe.

People who have a weak digestive system should not eat aloe.

American Ginseng 西洋参

Scientific name and origin: American ginseng is the root of the Araliaceae family. Latin name: *Panax quinquefolium* L. It is mainly grown in the US and Canada.

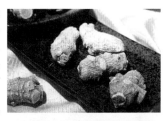

Properties and taste: Cool; slightly bitter and sweet

Channels of entry: Lung, heart, kidney and spleen

Composition and pharmacology: American ginseng is a functional herb with so many uses that you should always keep it on hand. It mainly contains quinquenoside-R1, ginsenoside-Ro, volatile oil and fatty acids. American ginseng strengthens qi and nourishes the

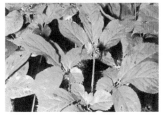

body, making it useful for recovering from illness, particularly lung ailments. It can also treat a number of other physical conditions as well as help in improving memory. Research shows that it helps the body cope with anxiety, regulates the flow of oxygen, reduces high cholesterol and fatigue, and promotes growth and development. It can regulate an irregular heartbeat, has anti-viral properties, and is helpful for those suffering from auto-immune diseases. American ginseng is also good for those that suffer from seizures, whether epileptic or as a result of high fever.

Culinary usage and medical applications:

1. Strengthening qi and nourishing yin: American ginseng is beneficial for the body after suffering from high fever, heavy

bleeding and heavy perspiration. It can boost memory, increase body fluid, alleviate fatigue, shortness of breath, vexation, excessive sweating, dry mouth, scanty and dark colored urine, and weak pulse.

2. Replenishing and restoring lung qi: Chinese people often use American ginseng after suffering from bronchitis or any kind of lung or respiratory diseases with symptoms of dry or bloody mucus cough and hoarse voice. People who have suffered for a few years from chronic conditions like tuberculosis can benefit from using American ginseng.

3. Strengthening lung and spleen qi, nourishing heart and stomach yin: It is also useful for heart qi and yin weakness (marked by palpitation, chest pain and pressure, and insomnia) or spleen and stomach qi and yin weakness (marked by poor appetite, abdominal distention and thirst).

4. Clearing away heat and promoting production of body fluid: It is useful for treating diabetes-related thirst, hunger and frequent urination, and weight loss.

How to eat?

American ginseng is easy to find, and can be used not only in teas but also on its own or as an ingredient in recipes. It is particularly beneficial for cancer of the nose and throat, and can be made into tea or eaten straight, as directed below.

1. Raw: Place one slice or 3g of American ginseng in the mouth, mix with saliva, and then chew slowly. This is beneficial for patients undergoing radiotherapy. Start consuming the ginseng about two weeks prior to treatment and continue until completed.

2. Tea: Make tea with one slice of American ginseng and 50ml of boiling water. Place the lid on the cup and let it steep for five minutes before drinking, eat the root after drinking the tea.

3. Decoction: Cook 3g of American ginseng with 100ml water. Bring it to a boil then let simmer for 30 minutes. Afterwards drink the water and eat the root. For those who do not like eating the root, the cooking time can be increased by 30 minutes to 60 minutes; then drink the liquid and discard the root.

4. Powder: Daily, mix 1–2g of the powder into any drink,

honey or yogurt.

5. Soup: Using 5–10g of American ginseng, 1 whole chicken or ½ duck and 1 liter of water, bring to a boil then simmer for 2 hours. (To reduce cooking time, use a pressure cooker for 15 minutes.)

Contraindication:

Do not consume American ginseng together with black false hellebores (*li lu* 藜芦) as this could prove toxic.

People with a weak digestive system who easily feel full or bloated, or have food allergies or intolerances should consume American ginseng with caution.

It is better not to drink any other types of tea, as tea contains tannins that disrupt the benefits of the American ginseng. After finishing the ginseng, wait three days before drinking other teas again.

Do not eat radishes while taking American ginseng, as they can reduce qi strength.

Apple 苹果

Scientific name and origin: Apple is the mature fruits of the Rosaceae family, with the Latin name of *Malus pumila* Mill. Apples are native to Europe and central Asia, and now can also be found in China's Hebei, Shanxi, Jiangsu and Shandong provinces.

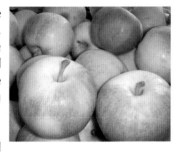

Properties and taste: Cool; sweet, acid

Channels of entry: Heart, lung and stomach

Composition and pharmacology: The apple's vitamin C protects cells from damage and supports healthy blood vessels. Eating raw apples cleans the teeth and massages the gums, which can ward off gingivitis. Quercetin, a common flavonoid and anti-oxidant found in apple skin (but not the pulp) has anti-inflammatory properties, which helps with conditions such as arthritis and prostate enlargement. Incorporating apples in your diet can help control insulin levels by slowing the release of sugar into the blood stream. This benefit is due to the presence of pectin.

Culinary usage and medical applications:

1. Increasing body fluid and cooling heat: Apples have both strengthening and regulating functions. They nourish body fluids and remove summer-heat, and help relieve restlessness, thirst and irritability.

2. Aiding digestion: Apples benefit the stomach, and help one sober up from alcohol. They treat lack of appetite, dry mouth, poor digestion, diarrhea and bloating in the abdomen after overeating or drinking too much alcohol.

How to eat?

1. Raw and juice: Eating a fresh apple or drinking apple juice daily is a great way to get vitamins. People drink apple and carrot juice to aid in achieving their ideal weight.

2. Jam: Apples often appear together with grapes in fruit jam but be careful that it doesn't contain too much sugar.

3. Dessert: Cooked or baked apple provides various choices of dessert.

4. Dried: For children do not like the texture of fresh apple, they can get its benefits from dried ones.

5. Wine: Apple wine is a good substitute for someone who cannot tolerate white or red (grape) wine.

Contraindication:

Do not consume too much because it can cause a greasy and tight feeling in the stomach or abdomen.

Asparagus 芦笋 (石刁柏)

Scientific name and origin: Asparagus is the tender sprout of Asparagaceae. The Latin name is *Asparagus officinalis* L. Northern Xinjiang produces wild asparagus; cultivated asparagus grow all over the China. The root also use as a medical herb.

Properties and taste: Neutral to cool; sweet

Channel of entry: Liver

Composition and pharmacology:
Asparagus is an excellent source of folate (along with vitamins B-6 and B-12). It is essential for a healthy cardiovascular system. It's also a very good source of potassium and low in sodium, a combination that provides a diuretic effect. Asparagus contains 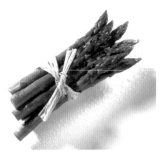 inulin, a type of carbohydrate that is favored by good bacteria in the intestinal tract. Asparagus contains more glutathione, a potent anticarcinogen and antioxidant, than other vegetables and fruits analyzed to date.

Asparagus is known to increase immune function and protect the liver.

Culinary usage and medical applications:
1. Cooling heat: It can cool the body and support production of bodily fluids to reduce thirst, irritability and dry skin. It treats psoriasis and hepatitis. It also treats leucopenia.

2. Relieving dampness: Asparagus can reduce both heat and damp, treat breast lump or mastitis.

How to eat?
Asparagus can be eaten fresh or dried. When using fresh, the quantity should be double that of dry.

1. Raw or juice: Eat raw asparagus as a component of a salad, typically as an appetizer.

Juice 500g of fresh asparagus and drink $^1/_3$ of the juice three times per day. Drinking this organic juice for 2 days can be beneficial for nose bleed or coughing dark mucus.

2. Steamed or stir-fried: Steamed or stir-fried asparagus can be incorporated into many dishes but be careful not to cook too long. For instance asparagus often stir-fried with chicken, shrimp, or beef, and also wrapped in bacon.

Asparagus is lightly steamed and eaten with oil or butter in US. Eating 60–90g in this way can cleanse and treat infections.

3. Stews or soup: The shoots are prepared also as an

ingredient in some stews and soups, i.e. vegetable soup or soup before meal.

Contraindication:

People who have a weak spleen or "cold stomach" should mix asparagus with garlic or only eat small amounts.

Astragalus Root 黄芪

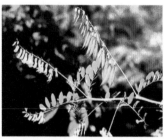

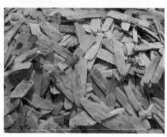

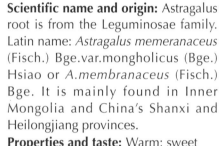

Scientific name and origin: Astragalus root is from the Leguminosae family. Latin name: *Astragalus memeranaceus* (Fisch.) Bge.var.mongholicus (Bge.) Hsiao or *A.membranaceus* (Fisch.) Bge. It is mainly found in Inner Mongolia and China's Shanxi and Heilongjiang provinces.

Properties and taste: Warm; sweet

Channels of entry: Spleen and lung

Composition and pharmacology: Targeting the spleen and lung, Astragalus root can be used when there are deficiencies of qi or blood in those systems. It contains astragalan, flavones triterpenes, alkaloid, glucuronic acid and microelements. It can strengthen both specific and nonspecific immunity, and improve hemopoiesis and synthesis of proteins. Its strengthening effect on the function of the sex glands can retard aging. At the same time, it has an impact on the two-way regulation of blood pressure and can protect the liver. Furthermore it can strengthen the energetic heartbeat, and prevent ulcers, viral myocarditis and inflammation as well as promote urination.

Culinary usage and medical applications:

Astragalus root has been used since ancient times both to treat illness and to stay healthy. It is susceptible to dampness and must be stored carefully.

1. Tonifying qi and lifting spleen yang: Treat qi deficiency of the spleen and stomach, manifested by (mental and physical) fatigue, poor appetite and loose stool. It can also counteract sinking of qi (digestive qi, middle-jiao qi) as manifested by constant diarrhea, or prolapse of anus or organs. Astragalus root can be used to remedy deficiency of both qi and blood, blood stagnancy due to deficiency of qi, and such symptoms as those manifested after stroke, facial paralysis, numbness and hemiparalysis. It is also used to treat diabetes due to deficiency of qi and body fluid (manifested by frequent thirst, hunger and urination) as well as chronic hemorrhage due to the weakness of spleen qi failing to control the blood.

2. Tonifying the lung and counteracting qi deficiency: Treat cough, asthma and shortness of breath due to deficiency of lung. It can counteract spontaneous sweating due to deficiency of resistance qi or consistent sweating after mild activity. It can also be used for flu due to qi deficiency (propensity to get the flu, aversion to wind, excessive sweating and prolonged course of disease).

3. Promoting tissue regeneration: Astragalus root can tonify the health qi and expel toxins. It can be used to treat boils, reproductive skin diseases, and swelling and ulcers on the body surface that are chronic. In these cases, according to TCM, the health qi is not strong enough to expel the toxin. Therefore tonifying the qi and blood can help stimulate cell and tissue regeneration, promoting healing.

4. Inducing diuresis to alleviate edema: Treat edema caused by qi deficiency; symptoms of shortness of breath, lassitude, water retention and reduced urination.

How to eat?

1. Tea or granule: Uncooked root is suitable for treating external diseases, and can function as a diuretic, which is always applied to spontaneous sweating, boils and edema. The cooked root is suitable for internal problems and can tonify spleen qi and lift yang. This has applications toward poor digestion, weakness of qi

and blood, as well as collapse of middle-jiao energy.

2. As herb and food: In ancient China, people not only treated illness with Astragalus root, but also used it to maintain health and strengthen the body. Astragalus root roasted with red dates, stewed with hen, or boiled with black beans are common formulas to strengthen senile and weak people, women after giving birth, and rehabilitation patients. If you consume Astragalus root regularly, it will increase your energy, improve your constitution, give you a rosy face and dewy skin, and enhance longevity.

3. Decoction: Use 15g for decoction, remove solids and drink the liquid, divided into 2 portions. It can benefit coronary heart disease due to qi deficiency of the heart, marked by angina, pale face, stuffy chest, shortness of breath or breathlessness during exertion, palpitations, whitish tongue or tongue coating, and weak or irregular pulse.

Contraindication:

The nature of Astragalus root is warm and tonifying. If you take too much, or if you do not have a weak and cold constitution, it may cause an excessive heat condition. It also stops sweating, so it is not suitable for those who are getting a flu, fever or stuffiness or distention in chest and belly.

For patients with tuberculosis, with fever, dry mouth and hemoptysis, it is not suitable for single use decoction.

Boils and ulcers in early stages should not be treated with Astragalus root.

Azuki Bean (Small Red Bean)　赤小豆

Scientific name and origin: Azuki beans (also spelled as adzuki or aduki) are seeds of the Lequminosae family. Latin name: *Vigna umbellata* (Thunb.) Ohwi et Ohashi and *V.angularis* (Willd.) Ohwi et Ohashi. *Vigna umbellata* grows in Zhejiang, Jiangxi and Hunan provinces. *V.angularis* grows all over China.

Properties and taste: Slightly cold to neutral; sweet and sour

Channels of entry: Heart, small intestine and spleen

Composition and pharmacology: Azuki bean contains triterpenoid saponin and azukisaponin 1 to 6. Azuki bean restrains male sperm.

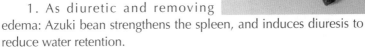

Culinary usage and medical applications:

1. As diuretic and removing edema: Azuki bean strengthens the spleen, and induces diuresis to reduce water retention.

2. Clearing heat and toxins: Azuki bean clears heat and toxic materials, and eliminates jaundice and boils (of the damp-heat type). It also harmonizes blood and drains off pus. Azuki bean can aid appendicitis, hemorrhoids, diarrhea or dysentery with blood in stools. It is used both internally and externally (ground into powder for external use in draining off skin pus).

How to eat?

1. Porridge: 90–150g Azuki beans, 50g rice, 3 cups water. Boil and stew into porridge (congee). Divide into 3 portions to eat over 3 days. Helps increase postnatal breast milk, improves count of platelets in the blood.

2. Steamed: 50g beans, 30g peanuts with peel. Wash beans and peanuts. Add 20g rock sugar and 3 cups water, and steam for 2 hours. Drink the liquid and eat the beans and nuts. Take for 15 days as a course against the tendency to bruise easily.

3. Soup: Boil 10–50g of beans as soup, divide into 2 portions to drink and eat. Use for 3 to 7 days to reduce pregnant edema. Combined with a low salt, high protein and vitamin-rich diet, this remedy is highly efficient.

4. Decoction: Decoct beans with other herbs.

Contraindication:

Eat with caution if you have a dry constitution.

Males should avoid eating in large quantities if he plans to father a baby.

65

Black Bean Sauce 淡豆豉

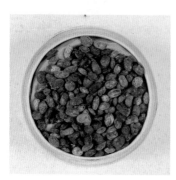

Scientific name and origin: Black bean sauce is produced from black beans after they have been steamed and fermented. Black beans are mature seeds of Leguminosae. Latin name: *Glycine max* (L.) Merr. Black bean sauce is produced in China's Jiangxi, Hunan and Jiangsu provinces.

Properties and taste: Neutral to cool; bitter and spicy

Channels of entry: Lung and stomach

Composition and pharmacology: Black bean sauce has soybean isoflavones, which can lower blood cholesterol and are thought to possess anti-cancer properties.

Culinary usage and medical applications:

1. Relieving the exterior syndrome: Black bean sauce can dispel the onset of the flu, sensitivity to cold or heat, or headache.

2. Relieving restlessness: Black bean sauce eases discomfort in the chest, palpitations, vexation and inability to fall asleep.

3. Helping circulation: Fermented black bean sauce (纳豆) can partially aid stroke recovery, lower blood lipids and prevent cardio-vascular disease.

How to eat?

1. Condiment: Black bean sauce is typically cooked with food such as fish or vegetables.

2. As an herb: Mix 9–12g black bean sauce with 3g of mint and green onion, and take during early onset of the flu.

Contraindication:

If the flu is already acute and accompanied by cold, use with caution.

If you experience weak stomach with nausea, use with caution.

Black Sesame Seed   黑芝麻

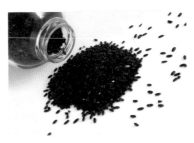

Scientific name and origin: Black sesame seeds are mature seeds of Pedaliaceae. Latin name: *Sesamum indicum* L.They are grown in all provinces of China.

Properties and taste: Neutral; sweet

Channels of entry: Liver, kidney, spleen and large intestine

Composition and pharmacology: Black sesame contains vitamin E, phytosterol, lecithin, pedalin, protein, potassium and phosphorus. Black sesame is also rich in omega 3 and fatty acids (oleic acid, linoleic acid, etc).Western medical research shows that black sesame has anti-aging properties. The high levels of omega 3 can lower high cholesterol, prevent hardening of the arteries, and reduce and stabilize blood sugar. Its fatty oils, especially vitamin E, strengthen and nourish the body, possess anti-inflammatory properties, and are good for detoxification.

Culinary usage and medical applications:

1. Nourishing liver and kidney yin: Black sesame can improve the quantity and quality of liver and kidney yin. It is beneficial for people who suffer from what TCM calls "weakness of the liver blood and kidney essence," characterized by low blood proteins, low oxygen levels in the blood, or poor circulation. Likewise, black sesame is good for poor liver or kidney functions. Some outward symptoms indicative of these internal weaknesses are premature whitening of the hair, hair loss, fatigue, losing teeth, dizzy spells, blurred vision and vision changes.

2. Relieving constipation by moistening large intestine: Black sesame is also very good for the large intestine as it can prevent constipation and hard stool. It is also helpful for people who are thirstier in the late afternoon or who feel hot in the early evening; this indicates dehydration and/or low grade fever.

How to eat?

1. With other foods, raw or cooked: Add some black sesame

seeds to stir fries, salad dressings, or other cooked dishes.

2. Snack and dessert: Black sesame powder can be made into a paste as the filling for Chinese sweet dumplings and moon cakes. Before making a powder, it is better to dry roast the seeds. The powder can also be mixed with lotus root powder to make a paste; honey or osmanthus flower is added for a sweeter taste. This is great as a snack or as part of breakfast. Many Asian supermarkets sell black sesame dessert powder in sachets; for an easy dessert, you only need to add boiling water. Other convenient snacks are crackers or nutrition bars containing black sesame. Usually black sesame is mixed with maltose sugar to help the sesame to stick to the bar.

3. As a drink: You can also make a warm drink by adding powdered black sesame, Chinese mulberries and boiling water to a cup and brewing for few minutes.

4. Porridge: Mix 100g of rice (presoaked for 20 minutes), 20g of black sesame, and 600ml of water, bring to a boil, then simmer for 45 minutes.

Contraindication:

People suffering from diarrhea should avoid consuming black sesame.

Clinical reports claim that in some rare cases, people have allergic reactions to black sesame. Symptoms include itchiness of the skin, cough, asthma attacks, perspiration, upset stomach, abdominal ache and nausea.

Consuming large quantities of raw black sesame can lead to obstructions in the intestines.

People who have kidney failure, and others who have been advised not to eat foods containing phosphorus, should consume only minimal amounts of black sesame.

Capsicum (Chili Pepper) 辣椒

Scientific name and origin: Capsicum is a fruit of Solanaceae, with the Latin name of *Capsicum annuum* L. Capsicum is indigenous

to the warmer regions of Mexico and
Latin America, and now grows all
over China, as well as many other
places in the world.

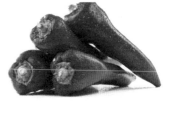

Properties and taste: Hot; spicy

Channels of entry: Stomach and
spleen

Composition and pharmacology: Capsicum has the highest
concentration of vitamin C of any vegetable. It also has vitamin
B, beta carotene, calcium and iron. The capsaicin in capsicum,
which is the addictive component that increases serotonin and
dopamine production, will give off feelings of happiness and con-
tentment.

Culinary usage and medical applications:

1. Warming the middle jiao, dispersing cold: Capsicum
can treat stomach aches belong to the cold type. It warms the
digestive system, notably the stomach, and can help stomach
ulcers. Capsicum is also noted for calming overactive qi, as
evidenced by hiccups, acid reflux or heartburn. For people who
don't like ginger, capsicum is a good alternative to fight off early
stage colds and coughs.

2. Increasing metabolism and fat burning: Capsicum has a
special mechanism that, combined with its fat burning nature,
tricks the brain into believing the body is not as hungry anymore.
If you can eat capsicum daily without adverse side effects, i.e.
people specifically with a cold constitution, 5–8g of capsicum
taken daily for 3 to 5 months can be an effective weight loss
supplement.

3. Improving appetite and promoting digestion: Capsicum is
good for lack of appetite, nausea and some type of vomiting.

4. Eliminating dampness: The root is particularly noted
for improving circulation to reduce swelling, hot feelings in
the muscles, lower back pain due to strain or over use, and
rheumatism.

5. Capsicum has anti-inflammatory properties as well,
especially on arthritic joints. It increases blood circulation,

especially in the cardiac region.

6. Capsicum can be rubbed directly on the skin to draw blood to that area, thereby improving circulation. Capsicum extract oil or patches may be available for skin application to improve blood flow to a specific area and reduce discomfort.

How to eat?

1. Stir-fried: Capsicum can be stir-fried with various vegetables or meats.

2. Sauce: It can also be made into sauce.

3. Oil: Capsicum oil is also very popular in China.

Contraindication:

As capsicum increases blood pressure, those who already suffer this condition should be careful how much they eat.

Similarly, anyone who is bleeding, especially internal bleeding or hemorrhoids, should not eat capsicum. Capsicum should not be used on existing rash-like skin conditions such as eczema, as it can aggravate it.

Those with certain constitutions, characterized by hot flashes, coughs, eye problems, eczema, dry constipation with excessive thirst, are not meant to eat capsicum.

Cassia Seed 决明子

Scientific name and origin: Cassia seeds are dried mature seeds of *Cassia obtusifolia* L., or in the smaller version, *C. tora* L. Cassia seed belongs to Leguminosea. While not originally from China, they are now produced all over China.

Properties and taste: Slightly cold; sweet, bitter and salty

Channels of entry: Liver and large intestine

Composition and pharmacology: Cassia seeds are thought to be an anti-bacterial. Cassia seeds can help clear up blurry vision, such as that caused by cataracts, as well as early stage night blindness. They are also noted for eliminating redness in the eyes caused by flu or pink eye.

Culinary usage and medical applications:

1. Cooling the liver and bringing shine to the eyes: Cassia seeds are known for their ability to cool the liver and kidneys. They can lower blood pressure and blood lipids, protect the liver, and aid bowel movement. They are used in cases of borderline high blood pressure, by those with family history of high blood pressure, or in the early stages of high cholesterol.

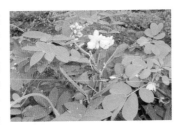

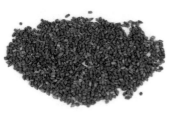

2. Moistening large intestine, increasing bowel movement: For people who have trained themselves to only have bowel movement once every 3–5 days, cassia seeds can correct this dangerous habit. Likewise, cassia seeds are used to aid bowel movement, especially in the presence of colon infection.

How to eat?

1. Tea: Make tea using 1 tsp whole or powdered cassia seeds. The same seeds can be used for multiple cups. Or use tea bags or a small package of granules emptied into the hot water.

For constipation with acne, bad taste in the mouth, combined with hot flashes but no stomach pain, cassia tea can increase bowel movements to once or twice per day. Take 15–30g of cassia seeds and 9g almonds, and make into tea, allowing the cassia seeds and almonds to soak open. If you prefer, you can add 1 tsp honey to your tea, and eat the almonds on the side instead.

2. Paste: Using whole cassia seeds, you can make a paste, adding honey for sweetness and to increase stickiness.

3. Decoction: For extended use of a month or more, a decoction may be more convenient. For acute conjunctivitis, make a decoction with 15g cassia seeds and 9g chrysanthemum, then take the mixture over 5 days. In the specific case of conjunctivitis combined with headache, choose small yellow chrysanthemum for additional potency.

4. Capsules or extract: Follow the recommended dosage on

the bottle.

Contraindication:

Cassia seeds are not advised for anyone with any of the following conditions: loose bowel movements, aversion to cold drinks, weak stomach.

Celery Stalk and Seed 旱芹

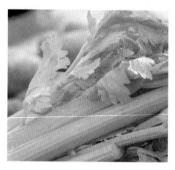

Scientific name and origin: Celery, including the whole root and leaves, comes from the Umbelliferae family. Latin name: *Apium graveolens* L. Celery grows all over China.

Properties and taste: Cool; sweet, spicy, slightly bitter

Channels of entry: Liver, stomach and lung

Composition and pharmacology: Celery contains phthalides, which can help reduce high blood pressure. Another compound in celery is coumarin, which may work to prevent cancer. Celery may lower cholesterol by increasing the secretion of bile. The main constituents of celery seeds are the characteristically-scented volatile oils such as d-limonene. Chemical components in celery include 3-n-butylphthalide, 3-n-butyl-4, 5-dihydrophthalide and coumarin. Celery is known for the following properties: reducing hypertension, anti-convulsion and anti-epilepsy. It has also shown promise in in-vitro studies as a good influence on learning and memory.

Culinary usage and medical applications:

1. Calming the liver and clearing away heat: Celery is used to cool heat and calm the liver. It can prevent dizziness and headache due to hypertension.

2. Expelling wind and removing dampness: Useful against carbuncles and swelling of the muscles.

3. Stopping bleeding and detoxifying: Helps with abnormal uterine bleeding and bloody stool.

4. Inducing diuresis: The diuretic function of celery helps to clear cloudy urination. It can reduce urgent, painful and frequent urination due to urethral inflammation. The seeds help to stimulate the removal of waste products from the body via the kidney and promote the flow of urine to flush the urinary system. These actions are useful in cases of arthritis, rheumatism and gout where the accumulation of acid in the body either triggers or irritates the condition.

How to eat?

1. Raw: Celery can be eaten fresh, for example, 30–60g of celery as salad with carrots.

2. Fresh juice: Drinking fresh juice made of 60g of celery can lower high blood pressure in its early stages.

3. Stir-fried: Stir-fry with lily bulb (do not cook for more than 5 minutes). This helps regulate liver qi and lung qi, and also cools body heat, calms the mind, and prevents mood swings.

4. Powder or decoction: Celery is an excellent cleansing food, TCM uses more fresh than dry. The dried roots and seeds are often applying as powder or decotion.

Contraindication:

People who have endogenous cold of the stomach and diarrhea should limit their consumption of celery, and eat with caution.

Cherry 櫻桃

Scientific name and origin: Cherries are fruits of the Rosaceae family. Latin name: *Cerasus pseudocerasus* (Lindl.) G. Don. The majority of edible cherries are derived from either *prunus avium* (the wild and sweet cherry) or from *prunus cerasus* (the sour cherry). China grows cherries in all regions.

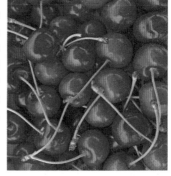

Properties and taste: Warm; sweet, sour
Channels of entry: Spleen and kidney

Composition and pharmacology: Cherries contain anthocyanins, the red pigment in the berries. In studies with rats, cherry anthocyanins have been shown to reduce pain and inflammation. Anthocyanins are also potent anti-oxidants, and are being actively researched regarding a variety of other potential health benefits. When eating a high-fat diet, cherries will reduce the possibility of weight gain or body fat buildup, thus preventing dysfunction in the heart and pancreas, also as shown in rats. Cherry also contains high levels of iron.

Culinary usage and medical applications:

1. Strengthening the spleen and stomach: Cherries improve the function of spleen, thus treating spleen weakness associated with dry mouth, lack of appetite and diarrhea. They also work to reduce lumbar and calf pain as well as numbness or palsy in the four limbs.

2. Nourishing the liver and kidney: Cherries help kidney deficiency associated with nocturnal emission, sore back and knees, and lack of energy.

3. Strengthening qi to nourish blood: By improving the quantity and quality of "spleen qi" and "original qi," cherries nourish the blood, thus moisturizing the skin to improve beauty, and help vertigo and palpitations.

How to eat?

1. Raw: Cherries can be eaten fresh or you can drink the juice, which is very good for stopping joint pain.

2. Cherry wine: Soak 500g of cherries in 750ml Chinese distilled liquor for a week. Cherry wine can prevent throat infections.

3. Dessert: Cherries combined with silver ear (a white fungus, see Silver Ear section for further description) makes a dessert that helps promote beautiful skin.

Contraindication:

Some constitutions cannot tolerate the iron and cyanogenic glucosides in cherries in large quantities.

If over-consumption occurs, make a soup with 200ml sugarcane juice and mung beans, drinking 200–500ml to detoxify.

Chinese Angelica Root 当归

Scientific name and origin: Chinese angelica is a root of Umbelliferae. Latin name: *Aaugellica sinensis* (Oliv) Diels. It is mainly produced in southeast Min County (Qinzhou), in Gansu province in China.

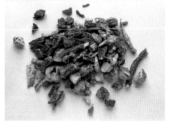

Properties and taste: Warm; sweet, pungent and bitter

Channels of entry: Liver, heart and spleen

Composition and pharmacology: Chinese angelica has volatile oil (ligustilide) and water solubility (ferulic acid), as well as polysaccharide, amino acid, vitamins and natural elements. It can strengthen both the specific and nonspecific immunity, and improve hemopoiesis. Furthermore, it protect the liver and is an anti-oxidant. It also acts against radiation, regulates heart rate, increases the flow of the coronary artery, reduces the oxygen consumption of myocardium, dilates vessels, brings down the peripheral resistance, prevents thrombus, and breaks down blood fat. It can be applied as a two-way regulator of uterine contraction, or to prevent inflammation, relieve asthma, induce analgesia, and in clinical tests, has been shown to fight germs and tumors.

Culinary usage and medical applications:

1. Tonifying the blood and promoting blood flow: Chinese angelica acts to tonify the blood, and it can also regulate blood circulation. It is effective in treating symptoms such as pale face, dizziness, vertigo, palpitation, poor memory, insomnia, fatigue and lassitude due to blood deficiency or the deficiency of both qi and blood. Furthermore, it is effective in treating numbness, tremors, stiff neck, and muscle weakness due to deficiency and stagnation of blood.

2. Regulating menstruation and alleviating pain: It can not only be used in promoting the blood flow to regulate menstruation, but also in tonifying the blood. It is one of the key herbs used in obstetrics and gynecology, and is widely applied in cases

of irregular menses, dysmenorrhea, amenorrhea, postpartum abdominalgia and uterine bleeding. However, it can be used to treat pains in all parts of the body, such as headache, abdominal pain, numbness with stiffness and spasm of limbs, and even for pain associated with injury as well as ulcers and sores induced by infection.

3. Loosening the bowel to relieve constipation: The nature of Chinese angelica is to nourish and moisten; therefore it can be used in treating dryness of the intestine due to blood deficiency, especially in a weakened older person and or someone with blood deficiency due to childbirth. Typical manifestations are weak, difficult excretion with dry stool, pale face, palpitation, shortness of breath, insomnia, memory problems and pale tongue with white fur.

How to eat?

1. Decoction: Use a slice of angelica (5–15g) together with other herbs. Put the angelica into an earthenware pot with 500ml of water to stew for 45 minutes, pouring off and reserving the liquid. Add another portion of water and cook again, adding this to the first batch of liquid, and stir well. Drink half in the morning and half in the evening for menstrual discomfort.

2. Medicated wine: Ancient records mention using angelica for medicated Chinese distilled liquor in treating arthralgia (joint pain).

3. Soup: Make a soup with ginger and mutton.

4. Powder: Angelica can be ground into powder for pills or applied as a facial mask.

Contraindication:

The nature of angelica is warm: Those who have yin deficiency in the stomach, lung yin deficiency with heat, kidney weakness with damp-heat, and liver-yang excess with phlegm-fire should use with great caution.

Chinese angelica should be used with care in cases of excess damp-heat, or damp-heat blocking the digestive system accompanied by loose stool.

Chinese Hawthorn Berry (Crataegus, Hawthorn Fruit)　山楂

Scientific name and origin: Hawthorn berries are mature fruits of Rosaceae. Latin name: *Crataegus pinnatifida* Bge. var.major N.E.Br. or *C. pinnatifida* Bge. The hawthorn berry comes from Henan, Shandong and Hebei provinces in China.

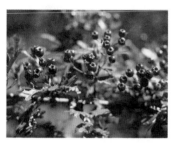

Properties and taste: Warm; sweet and sour

Channels of entry: Spleen, stomach and liver

Composition and pharmacology: Hawthorn berry contains hawthorn acid, tartaric acid, citric acid and flavonoids. Recent research shows that the hawthorn berry can strengthen the immune system, improve digestion, lower cholesterol, lower blood pressure, increase blood circulation to the heart, and contract the uterus. It also has anti-cancer, anti-inflammation and anti-oxidant properties.

Culinary usage and medical applications:

The Chinese hawthorn berry is tart, bright red and resembles small crabapples. They are used to make many kinds of Chinese snacks, including haw flakes and *tanghulu* (sugarcoated haws on a stick). The fruits are also used to produce jams, jellies, juices, alcoholic beverages, and other drinks.

1. Strengthening the stomach and aiding digestion: Hawthorn promotes digestion and removes stagnated food, so the most common TCM application is to alleviate indigestion. The hawthorn berry is particularly helpful in assisting the body to digest meat. When suffering from overeating, abdominal bloating or constipation with abdominal pain, one can first try eating hawthorn berries for relief before using other types of medication.

2. Promoting the movement of qi to relieve pain: Hawthorn berry can regulate qi movement in the stomach and colon to reduce or stop pain.

3. Activating blood circulation to dissipate blood stasis: It is

beneficial for women after childbirth if they experience pain in the lower abdomen, too much discharge, or painful menstruation. Women with menstrual cramps along with needle-like pain or blood clots benefit from eating hawthorn berries. Clinically, hawthorn berry can be combined with other types of Chinese herbs to treat uterine and ovarian cysts. Research shows that hawthorn products, especially extract, have helped patients with chronic heart failure, and is also beneficial in treating heart conditions. The hawthorn berry is good for blood circulation and in preventing blood clotting. Recently, the hawthorn berry was also found to reduce early stage high blood pressure, high cholesterol, and blood clotting in the major arteries.

How to eat?

1. Soup: Boil 60g fresh or 30g dried hawthorn berries, 20g of dolichos seeds (pre-soaked for 20 minutes), and 300–500ml of water, depending on desired consistency. Cook for 20 minutes. This soup is good for preventing indigestion, diarrhea, and abdominal pain.

2. Snack: Dried hawthorn can be eaten along with bananas to reduce constipation.

3. Tea: Boil 250ml of water. Prepare 5g of chrysanthemum flower, 10g of hawthorn berries, and 5g Chinese honeysuckle in a large cup or bowl; once the water has boiled, pour over the ingredients, put a lid on, and let brew for 10 minutes before drinking. This tea is very good for slimming and to reduce high cholesterol and high blood pressure in the early stages.

4. Powder: Grind 10g hawthorn berry and 10g green tea leaves into a powder. Make into tea, adding 2g to a cup of hot water. Drink 1 to 2 times per day to ease bloating in the stomach.

5. Porridge with hawthorn and millet: Bring 500ml water to a boil in a heat-safe ceramic pot. Add 5 pieces of sliced hawthorn berries (seeds removed) and boil for 30 minutes. Remove berries, add 100g millet and 3 tsp rock sugar, and cook for another 40 minutes.

6. Juice: Place 150g of fresh hawthorn berries in a juicer. Dilute the juice with 300ml water and then sweeten with 5 tsp honey. This juice helps fight fatigue and muscle soreness in calves and lower back.

7. Wine: Another way to treat the same symptoms is to add

some fresh hawthorn berries to a bottle of wine. Drink 20ml per day or eat one or two of the berries.

8. Boiled for various uses: Boil 30g of fresh hawthorn berries in 50ml of water for 5 minutes. Afterward, remove the berries but do not discard the water. Slice the berries and allow them to dry; to get out all the excess moisture a salad spinner can be used. Three berry slices can be made into a cup of tea or eaten as a snack. The cooking water from the berries can be used directly on the skin to alleviate itchiness.

Contraindication:

People who have stomach ulcers or high levels of stomach acid should avoid hawthorn berries or only consume with caution.

If you suffer from weakness of your stomach and digestive system or from diarrhea, you should also consume with care.

Overdose can cause cardiac arrhythmia and dangerously lower blood pressure. Milder side effects include nausea and sedation.

Chinese Raspberry 覆盆子（树莓）

Scientific name and origin: Chinese raspberries are fruits of the Rosaceae family. Latin name: *Rubus chingii* Hu. In China, they mainly grow in Zhejiang and Fujian provinces.
Properties and taste: Slightly warm; sweet and acid
Channels of entry: Liver and kidney

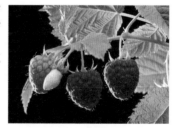

Composition and pharmacology: Raspberries contain anthocyanins, which have anti-oxidant and anti-microbial properties. Raspberries may also have cancer-prevention qualities. The high anti-oxidant power of raspberries makes them strongly recommended for preventing macular degeneration. Their very high fiber content may help prevent intestinal conditions, including constipation and hemorrhoids.
Culinary usage and medical applications:

1. Warming the body and strengthening qi and yang: Treat

male impotence and premature ejaculation, involuntary emission and nocturnal emission; watery vaginal discharge. Raspberries prevent and treat night and frequent urination.

2. Nourishing kidney and liver yin: It tonifies the organ system of the liver and brings shine to the eyes, decreases blurred vision, nourishes kidney essence, helps infertility, amenorrhea, and early grey and white hair.

How to eat?

1. Raw: Eat fresh or drink juice.

2. Tea: Drink 5–10g dried raspberries as tea, 5 times a week for 3 months to treat male sexual impotence, nocturnal emission.

3. Powder: Take 2g of raspberry powder with warm water to treat frequent urination. Or use mixed powder of raspberry 350g, wolfberry 500g, and mulberry 250g to warm the kidney system, and reduce spontaneously incomplete urination.

4. Pill: Take 240g wolfberry, 120g Chinese raspberry, and 60g Schisandra berry and roast lightly, then mix with honey to make pills. Pharmacies may also carry pills made of the berries along with a few herbal seeds.

5. Wine: Soak 300g of raspberries into 500ml of Chinese distilled liquor for 1 week.

6. Jelly: Use 500g of raspberries to make a jelly. Apply twice a year to bring a glow to the eyes and complexion. It also helps hair remain soft and elastic, and retain its original color.

7. External use: Juice 30g of fresh raspberry and spread on hair twice a day for a month to keep original color and moisture of hair.

Contraindication:

Do not take if you have body weakness with low grade fever.

Avoid eating raspberries if you are experiencing scant excreta and brown urine.

Chinese Yam   山药

Scientific name and origin: Chinese yams are roots of Dioscoreaceae, with the Latin name of *Dioscorea opposite* Thunb.

They mainly grow in Henan province and the Huai River area of China.

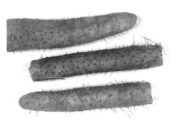

Properties and taste: Neutral; sweet

Channels of entry: Spleen, lung and kidney

Composition and pharmacology: Chinese yam contains diosgenin, dopamine, choline, amylon, glycoprotein, free amino acid, vitamin C, diastasum diastase and other compounds. Chinese yam has a double adjustment function in relation to colon motion and bowel movement, so it greatly assists digestion. It also helps to improve the immune system, reduces blood sugar, and acts as an anti-oxidant. Yam is a functional food that is good for sufferers of chronic diseases, such as diabetes, or a weak constitution.

Culinary usage and medical applications:

1. Strengthening the spleen and nourishing the stomach: Chinese yam can be used to treat low qi and yin of the spleen and stomach. This condition manifests in people who are very thin and often tired, with a poor appetite and loose stool. Fresh Chinese yam is a nutritious vegetable that can easily be digested, and thus it can be eaten over the long-term. It is the best food for people suffering chronic disease or weakness after a long illness. It is especially good for those who are under-nourished and for those with a weak digestive system.

2. Strengthening lung qi and nourishing lung yin: It is used to treat illness and pain in the patient's lung, including symptoms of fatigue, low and weak voice, weight loss, shortness of breath during exercise, thirst and so on.

3. Tonifying the kidney to consolidate the essence: Yams can also strengthen the kidney and improve kidney function, as in those with a deficiency of kidney qi and yin, with symptoms that include aching or weak knees, and frequent night urination. In males, symptoms may include spermatorrhea and premature ejaculation, while for women, watery vaginal discharge may be present.

4. Promoting the production of body fluid and benefiting qi: Chinese yams promote the secretion of body fluids and strengthen

qi, while reducing thirst, frequent urination, and recurring hunger caused by diabetes.

How to eat?

1. Steamed: Wash the fresh yam, then peel and steam. Mash it and then mix with lily bulb (optional) and press into small balls. This is good for the skin and nourishes the lung, for example treating tuberculosis and ailments inside the lung.

2. Powder: Using dried yams, pound into powder. Yam powder can be made into desserts. Suitable for consuming over a long period, it provides bodily strength to chronic disease sufferers.

3. Stir-fried: Fry with pre-cooked wheat bran or rice until the Chinese yam turns bright yellow. Fried yam strengthens the spleen when weakened by diarrhea.

4. Boiled or stewed: Boil 120–180g fresh Chinese yam for 20 minutes and eat for breakfast to control diabetes. Chinese yam can be also stewed with chicken, duck, or pork, and made into soup.

5. Decoction: Boil with other herbs to treat fatigue and loss of body essence.

Contraindication:

Do not take when suffering from indigestion, a full or bloated abdomen, poor appetite or when the tongue has a thick greasy coating.

Eating a high quantity (more than 200g) of Chinese yam could lead to intestinal distention.

Use great caution with raw Chinese yam as there have been reports of raw Chinese yam causing food poisoning.

Chive Seed 韭子

Scientific name and origin: Chive seeds are dried mature seeds of Liliaceae, with the Latin name of *Allium tuberosum* Rottl.ex Spreng. They are mainly produced in the Hebei, Shanxi and Jilin provinces of China.

Properties and taste: Warm; pungent and sweet

Channels of entry: Kidney and liver

Composition and pharmacology: Chive seeds contain nutrients such as amino acids, iron, manganese and zinc. Chive seeds can be taken for a wide variety of uses: to enhance sexual ability, as an anti-biotic activity, to repel insects, or remove damp phlegm.

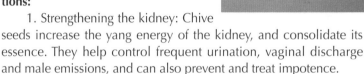

Culinary usage and medical applications:

1. Strengthening the kidney: Chive seeds increase the yang energy of the kidney, and consolidate its essence. They help control frequent urination, vaginal discharge and male emissions, and can also prevent and treat impotence.

2. Strengthening the liver: Chive seeds warm and strengthen the liver, improving the function of joints and tendons. They treat fatigue and weakness of the lower back and knees due to kidney and liver weakness.

How to eat?

1. Steamed: Use 3–9g of chive seeds, soaked thoroughly, and steam with 250ml water for 30 to 40 minutes. Drink the warm medicine, half in the morning and half in the evening, for children who are experiencing bed-wetting.

2. Powder: Grind 100g chive seeds into a powder. For one dose, drink 10ml of wine together with 6g of the powder; this will serve to strengthen the kidney's power, preventing emission.

3. Porridge: Prepare 100g of rice combined with 30g of chive seeds to treat vaginal discharge, frequent urination, and weakness of the lower back and knees.

Contraindication:

People who have a mixed dry and hot constitution should not take chive seeds.

Chrysanthemum   白菊花

Scientific name and origin: Chrysanthemum is a flower head

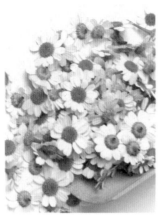

of the Asteraceae family. Latin name: *Dendranthema morifolium* (Ramat.) Tzvel. China's main supplies come from Anhui, Henan and Zhejiang provinces.

Properties and taste: Slightly cool; pungent, bitter and sweet

Channels of entry: Lung and liver

Composition and pharmacology: Chrysanthemum is anti-fungal and anti-bacterial, notably against bacillus. It can reduce fever, calm an overactive nervous system, and act as an anti-inflammatory. Chrysanthemum opens the cardiac artery and prevents spasms, while increasing oxygen flow to the heart to prevent high blood pressure.

Culinary usage and medical applications:

1. Dispelling onset of wind-heat: Chrysanthemum, when taken in the early stage of the flu, can reduce fever, headache, cough and susceptibility to bronchitis.

2. Relieving liver and internal heat: It also reduces red, itchy, light-sensitive, swollen eyes caused by allergies such as hay fever.

3. Helping cool summer-heat: It is a cooling drink in summer, and can treat red eyes and swelling gum in any season.

How to eat?

1. Tea: Chrysanthemum is primarily taken as a tea, by pouring boiling water (80–90 degrees) over 5g of dried flowers and steeping until they open for 5 minutes. As a cooling drink in summer, or to reduce eye irritation, enjoy the following tea: 10g chrysanthemum and 10g wolfberry. The tea can also be substituted for water in making small cakes.

2. Powder: Alternately, dried flowers can be powered and mixed with baking flour.

3. Decoction: Mix with other herbs to cook as a decoction. For example, 9g each of mulberry leaf and chrysanthemum are good for headache.

Contraindication:

People with bladder problems (too much or too frequent urine) should avoid chrysanthemum.

People with fatigue, diarrhea and cold feeling of stomach take chrysanthemum with caution.

Cinnamon Powder and Stick　肉桂粉 桂枝

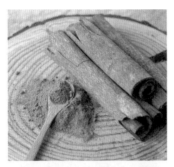

Scientific name and origin: Cinnamon powder and stick are ground bark and twigs, respectively, of the Lauraceae family. Latin name: *Cinnamomum cassia* Presl. In Asia, cinnamon is grown in Thailand, Vietnam and in China's Guangdong, Guangxi, Sichuan and Fujian provinces.

Properties and taste: Very hot (i.e. strongly warming); pungent and sweet

Channels of entry: Kidney, spleen, heart, and liver

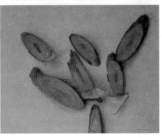

Composition and pharmacology: Cinnamon can improve cognitive skills, including memory and attention. Cinnamon contains volatile oils, cinnamic alcohol, cinnamic alcohol acetate, cinnamic acid, acetic acid, coumarin and tannins. Cinnamon counters the various side-effects of shrinking veins by opening them back up. It aids blood circulation and production, and is especially beneficial for the blood in the coronary artery and blood traveling to the brain. It is also a blood thinner. Cinnamon increases digestive enzymes and encourages peristalsis in the colon. It can restrain bacteria and fungus growth.

Culinary usage and medical applications:
Cinnamon Stick

Expelling cold: Cinnamon stick is used in TCM to expel the early onset of a cold. People who are averse to cold foods, drinks and environments can use cinnamon stick to warm those cold feelings in the chest and digestive track.

Cinnamon Bark Powder

Strengthening kidney yang: Due to its hot property, cinnamon is known for strengthening yang and vitality stemming from the kidney. In this case, those who would benefit from cinnamon usually suffer from lower back pain or cold in that region as well as the frequent need to urinate with little flow. Other signs specifically for men may be the tendency toward impotency or nocturnal emission, while women may have amenorrhea or show signs of infertility, and with children over 3 years old, bed-wetting may still a problem.

"Conducting the fire back to its origin": Conflicted symptoms, such as hot or flushed face combined with upset stomach after eating cold foods, also benefit from a small portion of cinnamon, 1–2g.

Subduing pain: Ground cinnamon, usually from the bark, is good for chronic pain as well as back pain, joint pain and menstrual cramps.

How to eat?

1. Powder: Cinnamon comes in a number of forms, including ground cinnamon, sold as a spice.

2. Bark oil: Cinnamon oil can be mixed into salad as part of a dressing or added on top of already cooked dishes for additional flavor.

3. Cinnamon stick: The stick comes from the tender branches of the tree. It can be added to stews or soup, being careful not to overcook.

4. Decoction: Cinnamon in its different forms can also be made into a decoction with other herbs. Some people have a cold stomach type of constitution, and have stomach pain or excessive saliva when they eat fruit in winter. To minimize negative reactions to cold, mix 3g cinnamon stick or 1.5g powder into tea and drink everyday for 5 days. For women who suffer menstrual cramps or pain, and abdominal distension or bloating, take 3g ground cinnamon and 20–30g brown sugar (optional) and drink as a tea twice a day, starting 2 days before menstruation begins. This drink is better in the winter or

for women who feel cold near menstruation time.

Contraindication:

Because of its blood thinning properties, cinnamon should not be consumed by people who are experiencing blood loss (for example, due to cough, hemorrhoids, etc.).

Due to the warming nature of cinnamon, people who have a fever, acute conditions indicating excess heat (sweating, rash, constipation), cold sores, or pimples on the back of the head are advised to avoid cinnamon.

Pregnant women shouldn't eat cinnamon too often; however, in cooking it is fine.

Clove 丁香

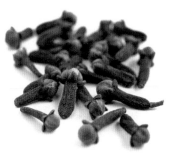

Scientific name and origin: Cloves are dried flower buds of the Myrtaceae family. Latin name: *Eugenia caryo-phyllata Thunb.* They are commonly imported from Tanzania, Malaysia and Indonesia. China's Guangdong and Hainan provinces also grow them.

Properties and taste: Warm; spicy

Channels of entry: Spleen, stomach, lung and kidney

Composition and pharmacology: Cloves contain eugenol, acetyl eugenol, clove enol, heptanone, α-clove ene, chavicol, benzyl alcohol and benzaldehyde. They can increase secretion of digestive juices to improve digestion, as well as reduce nausea, vomiting, pain and inflammation. If diagnosed with a dust mite infection, as determined by a blood test, one can take cloves to kill the mites. Cloves can act a blood thinner and encourage gall-bladder bile secretions.

Culinary usage and medical applications:

1. Counteracting cold: Cloves warm the stomach and gastric area, and calm upset stomachs, including easing nausea and hiccups.

2. Warming the kidney and strengthening kidney yang: To counteract low sex drive, brew cloves into tea.

3. Promoting qi movement: Cloves can be made into a rub to counteract pains in the side from exercise.

4. Counteracting diarrhea and feelings of cold in the stomach: Especially those that are common in infants and children.

How to eat?

1. Tea: Due to their warming nature, cloves can be used by pregnant women for morning sickness. They also can be used for stomach ailments. Mix 5g cloves and 5 greenish-yellow persimmon tops into tea, drinking 2 times per day for 3 days for hiccups and upset stomach, especially those caused by eating cold foods.

2. Powder: Ground cloves can be used as a spice in cooking.

3. As a rub: Mix 1 tsp ground cloves with honey or a thick lotion or other skin cream. Rub directly on the point of side pain that lingers after running or walking. Cover with a bandage and leave overnight or until pain disappears. This procedure can be repeated 2–3 times, and ultimately, this sort of side pain should disappear as soon as breathing recovers after exertion.

4. Whole cloves: They can be made into tea or added when steaming rice. For full medicinal properties, don't overcook.

5. On the skin: Put whole or ground cloves with cinnamon (optional) in a narrow cloth bag, and place the bag tightly over the belly button. The same pack can be used directly on the shoulder for frozen shoulder or as a pillow under the head for migraines.

6. Clove oil: It can be mixed with mint powder and applied directly on a toothache.

7. Decoction: Cloves can be boiled with other herbs for a decoction to treat problems with ovulation and hiccups.

Contraindication:

Similar to cinnamon, cloves should be taken with caution by people who have fever or other signs of having a hot constitution (internal heat).

Corn and Corn Silk 玉米 玉米须

Scientific name and origin: Corn is a seed of Poaceae. Latin name: *Zea mays* L.

Chinese medicine uses both the corn cob and corn silk. Corn grows all over China.

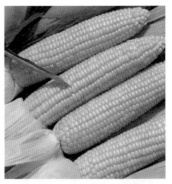

Properties and taste: Neutral; sweet (corn). Neutral; sweet, bland (corn silk)

Channels of entry: Stomach and large intestine (corn); kidney, urinary bladder, liver and gall bladder (corn silk)

Composition and pharmacology: Corn is composed of more than 60% starch, as well as fatty oil, vitamins B1, 2 and 6, and alkaloids. Corn is an anti-oxidant, which prevents aging and lowers blood sugar and lipids.

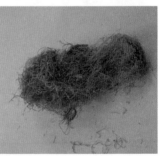

Corn silk contains gums, resins and vitamin C. Corn silk has a stronger diuretic function than corn. It also reduces hypertension.

Culinary usage and medical applications:

Corn

Strengthening and regulating middle-jiao: Corn awakens the appetite and is thus used to treat poor appetite.

Corn silk

Inducing diuresis and expelling swelling: Corn silk is used to treat cholecystitis, mastitis, diabetes and jaundice. It is used as a diuretic to reduce uncharacteristic swelling or summer swelling, to treat scant urine and urinary tract stones. Breathing in the smoke produced by burning dried corn silk can treat chronic sinusitis.

How to eat?

1. Boiled: Boil one ear of fresh corn with silk for 30 minutes, then eat the corn and drink the liquid, continuing for 3 days to prevent diabetes; repeat every 1–2 months. It also can be used to prevent miscarriage.

2. Stir-fried: Frozen corn is quick and useful to stir-fry with pine nuts and peas.

3. Corn flour powder: This can be used to make pancakes or corn porridge.

4. Decoction: To make a decoction using corn silk, use 30–60g fresh or 30g dried. Another recipe is useful in preventing diabetes: Bring to a boil 60g corn silk, 30g pearl barley, 30g mung beans, then stew for 45 minutes. Eat the pearl barley and mung beans, and drink the liquid.

Contraindication:

Eating too much fresh corn can disturb stomach function in people with a weak stomach.

Dandelion Root and Leaf　蒲公英

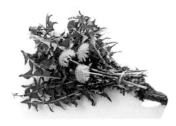

Scientific name and origin: Dandelions are roots and leaves of Asteraceae, with the Latin name of *Taraxacum mongolicum* Hand.acum mongo *T. sinicum* Kitag. They grow all over China.

Properties and taste: Cold; bitter, sweet

Channels of entry: Liver and stomach

Composition and pharmacology: The taraxasterol in dandelion may help against tumors. Research suggests that dandelion decoctions and infusions can stimulate the body's immune system and may have an anti-microbial function. Decoctions can act synergistically with certain drugs, for example sulfonamides, to increase their function.

Culinary usage and medical applications:

1. Cooling heat and expelling toxin: In a decoction, dandelion cools body heat, expels toxicity, and treats helicobacter pylori (HP positive).

2. Removing abscess and softening knots: A decoction can also dispel swelling, treating fibroadenosis of the breast, ovarian abscess and swollen prostate, as well as acne on the face and body. It also helps control the damp-heat kind of jaundice, urinary tract

infection and urinary bladder inflammation, as well as eliminating eye styes (of the heat type).

3. Treating the skin: For external use for rashes and lumps on the skin surface.

How to eat?

1. Raw: Eat as salad with other vegetables and fruit.

2. Tea: Dried or fresh dandelion can be drunk as tea with honey.

3. Powder: You can use dandelion and honeysuckle powder together to treat gastritis. Grind 30g dandelion root and 15g of honeysuckle into powder. Take 3g of the powder with honey, eat before breakfast and dinner, for a course of 10 days.

4. Decoction: Dandelion combined with hawthorn and Schisandra berry can reduce high blood lipids. Boil 15g dandelion leaf, 10g hawthorn and 5g Schisandra berry into a decoction. Drink 150ml as a dose, twice a day for 10 days.

Contraindication:

Overuse of dandelion can induce loose bowels.

Dolichos Seed (White Hyacinth Bean, Seed of the Lablab Vine) 白扁豆

Scientific name and origin: Dolichos seeds are mature seeds of Leguminosae. Latin name: *Dolichos lablab* L. Dolichos seeds are mainly grown in China's Jiangsu, Henan and Anhui provinces.

Properties and taste: Neutral; sweet and bland

Channels of entry: Spleen and stomach

Composition and pharmacology: Many vitamins and minerals are abundant in Dolichos seeds: fatty acids, protein, niacin, amino acids, vitamins A, B and C, alkaloids and saccharides. The seedcoat can strengthen and detoxify the immune system.

Culinary usage and medical applications:

1. Strengthening the spleen: Dolichos seeds nourish the spleen and balance the digestive system. They work to rectify low spleen qi, as characterized by weakness in the four limbs, poor appetite, and loose stool or diarrhea.

2. Dispelling dampness: They can also treat dampness and blockages of spleen qi, which lead to leukorrhea.

3. Eliminating summer-heat: Dolichos seeds dispel summer-heat and remove dampness, eliminating violent reactions such as vomiting and diarrhea. This condition is present when a person takes strong measures to avoid heat, such as always staying in cold environments, and drinking and eating only cold foods. Symptoms include high fever, sweating but failing to reduce heat, stuffy nose and thick nasal mucus, headache, dizziness, distention or swelling of the face and head, tiredness, thirst, irritability, difficulty urinating, and a thick yellow coating on the tongue.

How to eat?

1. Porridge: Boil 60g of Dolichos seeds, 100g of brown rice and 450ml of water together to make rice porridge. The function of this dish is to strengthen the spleen and stomach, clear away summer-heat, and reduce diarrhea. Adding 30g of Job's tears makes a porridge that is good for flu with body ache and headache.

2. Tea: Grind cooked Dolichos seed into powder, cut Chinese Mosla herb (香薷 , optional) into slices and place into a thermos cup, then add boiling water. Let soak for one hour. Drink this tea to prevent stomach flu and food poisoning in the summer.

Contraindication:

Dolichos seeds contain toxic proteins. Therefore fresh, uncooked seeds should not be consumed.

Fennel Seed and Fennel 小茴香

Scientific name and origin: Fennel seeds are mature dried fruit of Umbelliferae.Latin name: *Foeniculum vulgare* Mill. Fennel is found all over China, and it is easy to grow at home, so that you always have fresh fennel on hand.

Properties and taste: Warm; spicy

Channels of entry: Liver, kidney, spleen and stomach

Composition and pharmacology: Fennel seed contains volatile oil and aliphatic acid. It has been shown to aid digestive function, including improving secretion of gallbladder bile and liver tissue regeneration. Animal research has shown it tranquilizes pain.

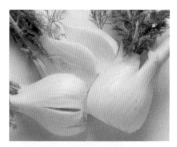
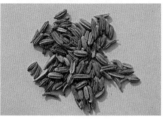

Culinary usage and medical applications:

1. Dispelling cold: Fennel seeds counteract cold, warming the internal body.

2. Regulating qi and stopping pain: Fennel seed eliminates abdominal pains, including those associated with hernias and menstrual periods. It can ease distention pain in the testes. Fennel seed also regulates the motion of stomach to prevent gas produced in the digestive system.

How to eat?

1. Condiment: Fresh fennel can be sprinkled on salad. The powder can be used to season dumpling fillings of meat or vegetables.

2. Tea: Stir-fry 30g fennel seed with 3g salt for 10 minutes. Use 3g of fennel seed for each cup of tea, taking it twice a day for 5 days. It can strengthen kidney qi.

3. Decoction: Fennel seed decocted with other herbs can be used to treat the cold type of hernia and stomach ache.

Contraindication:

People with a mixed dry and hot constitution should avoid eating it.

Fenugreek 胡芦巴子

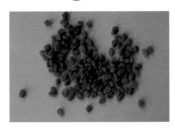

Scientific name and origin: Fenugreek is a seed of Leguminosae. Latin name: *Trigonella foenumgraecum* L. They are grown in China's Jiangsu, Shandong, Anhui and Shaanxi provinces.

Properties and taste: Warm; bitter

Channels of entry: Liver and kidney

Composition and pharmacology: Fenugreek is composed of quercetin, trigonelline, choline, diosgenin, and vitamin B1. These components can prevent and treat diabetes and ulcers, and are also thought to have anti-cancer properties.

Culinary usage and medical applications:

1. Warming kidney yang and strengthening kidney essence: Fenugreek helps impotence (ED).

2. Dispelling cold and dampness, stopping pain: It prevents and treats lower back weakness when associated with a cold feeling, or sinking feelings in the lower back or abdomen. It is also used to treat hernia pain, aversion to cold, and abdominal distention.

How to eat?

1. Powder: Grind it into a powder, and mix with cereal grains.

2. Tea: Drink fenugreek mixed with fennel as a tea for kidney deficiency of lumbago.

3. Decoction: To treat kidney weakness as evidenced by seminal emission, frequent need to urinate, or wetting oneself easily, make the following decoction: Bring 15g fenugreek and 15g raspberry to a boil, then simmer for 30 minutes. Drink the liquid twice a day for a week, mixing with warm rice wine. To treat hernia of the small intestine with a cold feeling and abdominal pain, try this decoction: Bring 15g fenugreek and 6g fennel to a boil, then simmer for 30 minutes. Drink the liquid twice daily for 3 days. It also warms and alleviates pain.

Contraindication:

Those with a dry constitution, with symptoms including thirst, hot flashes and heavy sweats, should only use fenugreek with caution.

Fig 无花果

Scientific name and origin: Figs are fruit of the Moraceae family. Latin name: *Ficus carica* L. They mainly grow in western Asia and in southern areas of China.

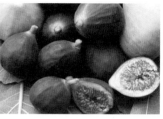

Properties and taste: Neutral to cool; sweet

Channels of entry: Lung, stomach and large intestine

Composition and pharmacology: Figs contain high citric acid, fig polysaccharide, saponin and glucoside compounds. Figs can enhance cellular immunity and reduce susceptibility to some cancers. They also have analgesic properties.

Culinary usage and medical applications:

1. Nourishing and moisturizing: Figs offer gentle nourishment and moisture for the digestive track.

2. Reducing heat: Figs cool heat, increase production of body fluids, aid appetite, dispel swelling and detoxify food poison. They can treat hemorrhoids, sore throat, hoarseness of voice and dry cough.

3. Aiding digestive system: Figs induce breast-milk, eliminate parasites, dispel swelling and burning sensations, and stop diarrhea and dysentery.

4. Treating skin externally: To treat vitiligo.

How to eat?

1. Fresh: Take two fresh figs on an empty stomach to treat hemorrhoids with swelling pain accompanied by bleeding. Take twice a day, continuing for three days for best results. Take 5 fresh figs or 20g dried fig after a meal for 2 weeks to prevent or treat stomach and colon cancer.

2. Soup: To prevent and treat cancer of the esophagus, take 500g of fresh fig, 100g of lean pork meat, and stew for half hour. Drink the soup and eat the meat for a month as a course of treatment.

3. External: Slice 250g of fig fruit and leaves, soak into 50%

alcohol for 7 days. Use to treat vitiligo, brushing the solution on the affected area, continuing for 2 weeks.

Contraindication:

If one's stomach is adverse to cold drinks or feels cold pain easily, eat figs with caution.

Flaxseed (Linseed)　亞麻子

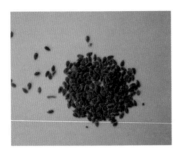

Scientific name and origin: Flaxseeds are the mature seeds of the Linaceae, with the Latin name of *Linum usitatissimum* L. China's northern and southwestern regions grow flaxseeds.

Properties and taste: Neutral; sweet

Channels of entry: Lung, liver and large intestine

Composition and pharmacology: Flaxseeds reduce cholesterol and triglyceride levels. Ground flaxseeds provide fiber that can reduce cholesterol levels in people who have atherosclerosis and heart disease. The magnesium in flaxseeds can lower high blood pressure and help in the treatment of insomnia. Flaxseeds contain lignans substance, which protects against the development of breast cancer in women. Flaxseeds can also regulate the body's response to inflammation.

Culinary usage and medical applications:

1. Nourishing blood and body fluids: Due to these properties, flaxseeds can address the condition wherein the skin itches in different places in succession. To heal skin cracks caused by psoriasis or eczema, eating flaxseeds can be useful.

2. Strengthening the liver and kidney: To aid recovery from severe diseases and alleviate weakness, flaxseeds are taken long term (about 3–6 months). Flaxseeds are thought to regenerate the spongy tissue of the brain, which is believed to be produced in the kidney. They can also alleviative unexplained mild vertigo. The estrogen in flaxseeds can reduce menopausal symptoms such as hot flashes or mood swings.

3. Moistening dryness and eliminating constipation: Flaxseeds are also advised for people, typically the elderly, who have constipation caused by dryness and weakness. They prevent and treat dry feelings in the body as well as constipation.

4. External use: Ground flaxseeds or flaxseed oil can also be applied topically for problems including canker sores, vaginal pimples, or pimples on the top of the head, especially found in children.

How to eat?

1. Mixed with other food: In order to benefit from the properties of flaxseeds, they must be soaked overnight before use or else ground (such as with a blender) to release the oil contained inside the shell. For example, if adding them to fruit smoothies, first blend the flaxseeds alone in the blender, then add the fruit, liquid and other ingredients.

2. Steamed: Flaxseeds, steamed and then crushed and mixed with honey, can be eaten by post-partum women to address symptoms of dryness, constipation, weakness and hair loss.

3. As an herb: Consuming a 3-month course of flaxseed can be used to prevent hardening of the arteries caused by high cholesterol and borderline high blood pressure. Consume 12g (either as one dose, or split among 2 doses) of flaxseeds daily, continuing for 3 months.

4. Decoction: Flaxseeds cooked with angelica root can treat dry and cracked skin.

Contraindication:

Those prone to diarrhea should avoid taking too many flaxseeds. After 15 days of continuous usage, a 3-day break should be taken. Furthermore, after 3 months of ongoing usage, a break of about 15 days is necessary.

Garlic 大蒜

Scientific name and origin: Garlic is a bulb of Liliaceae. Latin name: *Allium sativum* L. Garlic grows all over China.

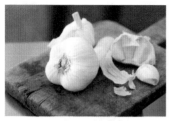

Properties and taste: Warm; spicy
Channels of entry: Spleen, stomach, lung and large intestine
Composition and pharmacology: The benefits of garlic are plentiful. Aged garlic extracts may prevent dementia by protecting neurons in the brain, and thus help fight cognitive decline and improve memory. There is convincing evidence that garlic can help prevent cancer of the stomach and colon. A substance called dially1 disulfide, found in garlic, appears to ward off carcinogens produced by meat and fish cooked at high temperatures. Garlic works against anti-microbial infections, bacteria, virus, fungus and irregular heartbeat, as well as reducing blood lipids and atherosclerosis, and thinning the blood. Garlic has anti-tumor, anti-oxidant, anti-free radical, and anti-mutation properties. It protects the liver from invasion by viruses, and mends the dynamic balance of the immunity system.

Culinary usage and medical applications:

1. Promoting movement of qi: Garlic warms the digestive system and moves body qi. It treats food retention, cold sensations and pain in the abdomen, and diarrhea.

2. Dispelling toxic materials: Garlic detoxifies, kills parasites, and inhibits the flu virus, tuberculosis, dysentery and vaginal discharge. It also helps reduce swelling and edema.

3. Treating fungal infections: Garlic juice can be applied topically on the affected area to treat fungal infection of hands, and itchiness, especially due to athlete's foot.

How to eat?

1. Raw or juice: Peel off the skin, slice the garlic, and eat after 15 minutes of oxidation, taking 2 pieces each time. Or slice and toss into salad as a seasoning. Remove any breath odor by drinking yogurt.

2. Steamed: Garlic tastes delicious when steamed with shrimp or fish.

3. Stir-fried: Garlic stir-fried with broccoli and snow peas is a tasty dish, popular in Shanghai. It also reduces cold properties in food.

4. Pickled: Garlic soaked in vinegar makes a suitable pickled appetizer.

5. Soup: Garlic goes well with mixed vegetable or meat soups.

Contraindication:

People who have a mixed dry and heat constitution should not take garlic.

People with infectious illness should avoid raw garlic, and be cautious with cooked garlic.

When people suffer from mouth, eye or tongue diseases, they should avoid raw garlic.

Ginger and Dried Ginger   生姜干姜

Scientific name and origin: Ginger and dried ginger are fresh or dried roots of the Zinziberaceae family. Latin name: *Zingiber officinale* Rosc. The provinces of Shandong, Sichuan, Guangdong and Guangxi produce most of the ginger in China.

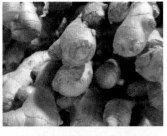

Properties and taste: Warm; slightly spicy (fresh ginger). Hot; spicy (dried ginger)

Channels of entry: Lung, spleen and stomach (dried ginger also targets the kidneys and heart)

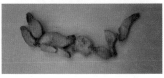

Composition and pharmacology: Ginger aids digestion, protects the stomach lining, and reduces vomiting and nausea. It is also an anti-oxidant and has anti-aging properties, and protects the liver and gallbladder. Ginger, when consumed in large quantities, counteracts the toxins from fish or mushrooms that can lead to food poisoning. To lower fever, ease pain, and reduce inflammation, ginger is beneficial. It moderates both high and low blood pressure. As a relaxant from panic or high-anxiety situations, ginger is useful. Ginger can also lower cholesterol and reduce fatty liver.

Culinary usage and medical applications:
Fresh ginger

1. Expelling onset of cold, relieving phlegm to stop cough: Fresh ginger aids in the release of cold, both the cold virus and sensations of cold, sometimes characterized by failure to sweat.

2. Warming digestive system to strengthen stomach and eliminate vomiting: A simple drink of ginger water can cure hiccups. To ease motion sickness or morning sickness in pregnant women, ginger tablets or ginger tea are a good alternative to medications. Dried ginger also treats stomach pain, gastric disorder causing nausea regurgitation, and diarrhea.

Dried ginger

1. Warming the body and expelling internal cold: Treat feelings of cold in the limbs and up the back.

2. Warming the lung and digestive system: Dried ginger helps limit sputum in the stomach that causes abdominal cold pain, vomit and diarrhea; and watery phlegm in the respiratory system, causing cough and asthma.

3. Strengthening yang and easing circulation: It helps against painful joints and heavy and numb feelings in the four limbs. Ginger can even be made into a poultice and applied directly on the joints for joint pain.

How to eat?
Fresh ginger

1. Tea: When cold feelings overtake the body in cold rain, snow, or when being exposed to cold air after sweating, make the following recipe and immediately after drinking, go to bed with lots of blankets to sweat out the cold: Bring 3–5g brown sugar, 5g ginger, and water to a boil; drink a large cup while still hot.

2. Raw or Juice: Ginger can be pressed into a liquid and made into a drink, used to treat morning sickness or vomiting.

3. Mixed with cloves: If food remains undigested and leads to sensations of nausea or regurgitation after 1–2 days, try this recipe: Press the ginger to produce a liquid and mix with ground cloves, use resulting mixture on top of any food. Or boil ginger with whole cloves into a tea. This recipe is also suited to people who are averse to cold.

3. Stir-fried and soup: Ginger is great in vegetable stir-fries or meat soup.

Dried ginger

1. Candy: Candied ginger is a good snack.

2. Herb tea: To open the heart meridian and warm kidney yang, as when blood pressure and blood sugar fall too rapidly, make 10g dried ginger, 5g cinnamon stick and 3g ginseng (optional) into tea.

3. Powder: Ginger powder can made into a drink, or mixed with other herbs for a decoction to treat stomach cold pain.

4. Tablets: Ginger tablets can prevent motion sickness.

5. External use: For a recipe to treat joint pain, slice 60g dried ginger and crush 30g dried chili, and put into a pot with 1L water. Bring to a boil and then simmer for 40 minutes. As it is simmering, use the heat to first steam the joint. Next absorb the liquid with a thick cloth, and place the hot cloth over the joint for 20 minutes. Pre-mixed skin application packages of ginger with chili and mixed herbs may also be available.

Contraindication:

People who are constantly flushed, suffer hot flashes, or have high fever or long-term low-grade fever should not eat too much ginger.

Due to its warming nature, people who are already hot should not eat ginger. Dried ginger is not advised for people who are coughing or vomiting blood or have any other signs of bleeding.

Gingko Nut   白果

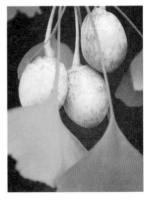

Scientific name and origin: Gingko nut is a mature seed of Ginkgoaceae. Latin name: *Ginkgo biloba* L. Gingko nuts are grown in all provinces of China.

Properties and taste: Neutral; sweet, bitter, astringent

Channels of entry: Lung and kidney

Composition and pharmacology: Gingko nuts contain a variety of nutrients, including starch, proteins, adipose carbohydrate, as well as vitamins and minerals, such as vitamins C and B2, beta carotine, calcium, phosphorous, iron and potassium. Gingko also contains micronutrients such as ginkgoicacid, bilobol and polycose. Gingko nuts can slow the aging process, improve cerebral ischemia, expel phlegm, reduce hypertension, suppress over-active immune response, and help generate both an anti-allergic and anti-microbial reaction.

Culinary usage and medical applications:

1. Restraining lung qi: Gingko nuts can enhance lung qi, and with their astringent and bitter properties, they can relieve cough, ease wheezing, and expel phlegm. They can also relieve shortness of breath and reduce the volume of sputum to aid treatment of bronchitis and asthma. Symptoms of such a condition may include wheezing, cough, shortness of breath when lying down, and cyanosis (blue color from lack of blood oxygen) in lips and nails.

2. Arresting leukorrhea and polyuria: Gingko nuts are also effective at stopping vaginal discharge and excessive urination as caused by weakness in the spleen and kidney. Gingko is an effective functional food for preventing and treating leukorrhea (profuse discharge), chronic urine infection, enuresis (bed-wetting), and frequent need to urinate.

How to eat?

1. Boiled: Peel off the outer shell, and then bring 10 gingko nuts to boil in 75ml of water for 10 minutes. Drink the liquid and eat the nuts. Sweeten with sugar or honey, if desired. This can prevent or treat ordinary cough, shortness of breath, or cough due to tuberculosis. Someone who suffers from a chronic weakness in the body should eat 8 to 12 gingko nuts per day for 1 month as food therapy.

2. Powder: As a remedy for diarrhea caused by a poor diet: Crush 2 gingko nuts into powder, then put the powder into a small hole created on the surface of an egg. Eat one of these eggs, steam until well done, daily to alleviate indigestion along with loose stool.

Contraindication:

Eating a large quantity of raw gingko nuts can create a toxic buildup, especially in children.

Gluey Millet 秫米

Scientific name and origin: Gluey millet comes from seeds of the Poaceae, with the Latin name of *Setaria italica* (L.) *Beauv*. It is known by a variety of other names, including foxtail millet, Italian millet, German millet, Hungarian millet and Japanese millet. It is grown in northeastern China as well as Shandong and Hebei provinces.

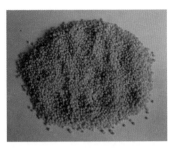

Properties and taste: Cool; sweet
Channels of entry: Lung, stomach and large intestine
Culinary usage and medical applications:

1. Aiding digestion and calming the mind: Gluey millet strengthens weak digestive systems and improves insomnia due to indigestion.

2. Moisturizing the body: Gluey millet is a yin tonic, helping to moisturize the whole body, including the skin. For post-partum women, millet is thought to increase breast milk production.

3. Dispelling wind and eliminating dampness: It reduces rheumatism, spasms and sore or aching muscles, especially those related to cold or wet environments.

4. Detoxifying and relieving skin rash: The cooling properties of millet are good for children when they have a heat rash.

How to eat?

1. As rice or thick soup: Millet is typically taken before a meal or before bedtime to improve digestion and aid sleep. To improve sleep, millet can be made into a soup or porridge. Millet can sometimes be used instead of rice as a staple grain.

2. Snacks: It can also be made into dry, crunchy snacks when mixed with sugar and peanuts.

3. Flour: If ground millet, made into flour, is available, it can be used to make pancakes or as a general substitute for white flour.

4. Wine: Millet can be fermented following the same process as beer or cider to produce an alcoholic drink.

5. Decoction: Gluey millet can be mixed with pinellia rhi-

zome and cook as a decoction to prevent insomnia.

Contraindication:

Eating millet once a day, normally 9–15g (and no more than 30g), is sufficient.

Children who lack an appetite cannot eat gluey millet often.

Grape 葡萄

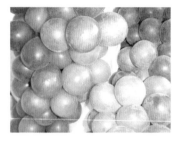

Scientific name and origin: Grapes are mature fruits of the Vitaceae family. Latin name: *Vitis vini fera* L. While originally grown in west Asia, now various regions in China also grow grapes.

Properties and taste: Neutral; sweet and acid

Channels of entry: Lung, spleen and kidney

Composition and pharmacology: Grapes contain the polyphenol tannin, which scientists discovered can destroy or hinder viruses, including the HIV virus. Grape seeds also have the potential to reduce bad cholesterol levels and help prevent atherosclerosis according to a 2007 study from Japan. Researches find that purple grape juice and wine are helpful in preventing the development of cardiovascular disease. Grapes, except the white grape, contain resveratrol, which may serve as an anti-oxidant. Grapes also have anti-cancer and anti-aging properties. They protect and prevent liver damage and prevent an antagonistic immune system.

Culinary usage and medical applications:

To get maximum health benefits, one should eat the entire grape, including skin and seeds. As a medical plant, the dried cultivated fruit, root, stem and leaf of wild grapes are all used.

1. Nourishing qi and blood: Grapes and grape wine (in small quantity) improve the quantity and quality of qi and blood, strengthening and nourishing the body. They reduce dizziness, palpitations and night sweats. Grapes also calm the mind and stop

vomiting and stomach pain. Furthermore, grapes help chronic cough from weak lungs, and backache due to weak liver and kidney.

2. Strengthening tendons and bones: The root and stem of grapes benefit tendons and ligaments, and treat chronic arthritis.

3. Inducing diuresis: The root and stem of grapes increase urine, and aid with difficult urination and edema.

How to eat?

1. Raw: Fresh grapes or grape juice. To improve anemia accompanied by dizziness, palpitation, and tiredness, drink 50ml of juice, 2–3 times per day.

2. Dried: Dried grapes (raisins) mixed into oatmeal or yogurt are a good breakfast or snack.

3. Wine: High quality wine from grapes is now produced in many countries and is widely available. We can only get the healthy benefits by drinking a small quantity of wine.

4. Extract: Grape extract can be use as a food supplement for hay fever.

5. Decoction: The root and stem of grapes combined with other herbs increases urine.

Contraindication:

Use with caution if you are experiencing any of the following: feeling hot, dry and weak; heartburn and constipation; nausea; or an accumulation of yellow phlegm.

Eating too many grapes can cause internal heat with symptoms of irritability and poor eyesight.

Green Tea 绿茶

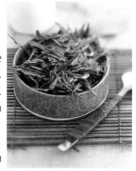

Scientific name and origin: Green tea is made from tender leaves or shoots of Theaceae, with the Latin name of *Camellia sinensis* (L.). China's Sichuan, Anhui, Fujian and Yunnan provinces are its native regions.

Properties and taste: Cool; bitter and sweet

Channels of entry: Heart, lung, kidney and stomach

Composition and pharmacology: Green tea is effective in reducing the buildup of dental plaque, which helps prevent the development of gingivitis. New research indicates that epigallocatechin gallate (EGCG) and the amino acid L-theanine found in green tea may help improve memory and learning. Several studies indicate that the polyphenols in green tea protect dopamine neurons, which are involved in Parkinson's disease. Green tea contains some caffeine, acting as a general stimulant. It reduces blood pressure and blood sugar, and increases urine. Green tea also has anti-cancer properties.

Culinary usage and medical applications:

1. Clearing heat and toxicity, refreshing the body: Green tea clears the eyes and head, and aids concentration and alertness. It is known to reduce hot feelings in the body manifested as dizziness, thirst and irritability.

2. Aiding digestion: Especially after a heavy meal, green tea is good for relieving food stagnation, poor digestion and damp-heat diarrhea, and for reducing the food's conversion to and storage as fat. Some people, primarily those who have a hot constitution, can use green tea as a hangover cure.

3. Energizing the body: Green tea is a good alternative to coffee for caffeine to aid waking and generate early morning energy. Specifically, early morning tiredness may be caused by blockages in energy flow, which green tea helps to eliminate.

4. Treating phlegm and bad breath: Conditions commonly found in smokers—daily morning phlegm or mucus, or persistent bronchitis, also known as damp constitution—usually find relief through drinking green tea. Green tea, including chewing the brewed leaves, is noted for masking bad breath.

5. Inducing diuresis: Green tea increases urination, helps dark colored urine, oliguria (low output of urine) and edema.

How to eat?

1. Tea: Green tea is most commonly consumed simply as a hot drink. Avoid bottled green tea drinks, because sugar or preservatives may be added, thereby changing the properties of the tea. You should follow the old Chinese saying: "Do not drink overnight

tea." Likewise, don't add milk or sweeteners because they alter the active properties.

2. Eggs: If you need to use up older green tea leaves, you can make flavored boiled eggs. Wash eggs and place them in a stove-safe earthenware container along with water and tea leaves. Simmer, lid on, for 5 minutes. Then slightly crack the top of the eggs to allow more flavors to enter. Continue simmering for another 15 to 25 minutes.

3. Extract or powder: Green tea capsules, extract, powder and tea bags are also available.

4. Decoction: Tea mixed with lotus leaves can be used for weight reduction.

Contraindication:

Green tea should be avoided by people who have a "cold or weak" stomach and/or digestive system.

People who have insomnia or constipation should not drink tea.

Avoid drinking tea when eating ginseng, poria or iron.

Honey   蜂蜜

Scientific name and origin: Honey is the gooey substance of the Apidae family. Latin name: *Apis cerana* Fabr., or *A. mellifera* L. Honey is produced all over China.

Properties and taste: Neutral; slightly sweet

Channels of entry: Lung, spleen and large intestine

Composition and pharmacology: Honey stimulates the regeneration of tissue and mucus. It can reduce blood pressure and open the veins close to the heart. It eases upset stomach by reducing acidity, and also reduces toxins.

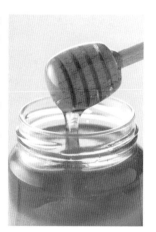

Culinary usage and medical applications:

1. Strengthening the body: Honey is good for general weakness, muscle soreness and narrowing of blood vessels, particularly common in winter. Women who are feeling irritable, as well as uncharacteristically hot or dry, should eat honey.

2. Strengthening digestion: Honey fortifies the digestive tract, moistens, relieves stomach spasms, treats stomach ulcers and eases hunger pains, stomach ache and rhinorrhea (runny nose) with turbid discharge.

3. Nourishing the lung: Honey strengthens lung qi, nourishes the lung to stop cough, especially chronic dry cough accompanied by shortness of breath, fatigue and dry throat, and helps clear the throat of mucus.

4. Moistening the colon: Honey is beneficial to the large intestine as it eases constipation, when mixed with water and taken either orally or administered directly to the colon. To ease constipation and dry skin, use the recipe listed under "silver ear," substituting honey for brown sugar.

5. Clearing toxins: To reduce swelling and itching caused by bug bites, honey can be applied directly on the skin. It also removes aconitic toxicity.

6. Treating burns. Honey, used externally, can treat scalds and burns.

How to eat?

1. Sweetener: Honey is a healthy natural sweetener that can be added to drinks, such as tea, or even used instead of jam on toast. To treat stomach ulcers, consume 20g of honey per day, such as before bed.

2. As a drink: For constipation, add ground 4–5 almonds and honey to water. If the almonds are too hard, they can be boiled soft. Using a special type of honey made from the flowers of the Japanese Pagoda tree is good for reducing bleeding from hemorrhoids.

3. Paste: Honey can be mixed with powdered herbs to make a beneficial herbal paste.

4. Steamed: Honey steamed with pear treats dry cough.

5. Soup: For a quick soup, honey together with eggs treats abdominal pain and nausea, or with sweet almond soup, reduces

dry cough.

6. Decoction: 30–60g of high dosage honey, mixed with other herbs, can be used to treat stomach ulcer.

7. Herbal Medicine: It can be found as an ingredient in pills or soft extracts of many Chinese patent and external use medicines.

Contraindication:

While honey is good for the digestive system, when experiencing bloating, diarrhea or abdominal distention, it should be used with caution.

Honeysuckle　金银花

Scientific name and origin: Honeysuckle is a fresh or dry flower bud of Caprifoliaceae. Latin name: *Lonicera japonica* Thund., *L. hypoglauca* Miq., *L. confusa* DC. and *L.dasystyla* Rehd. They grow in China's Henan and Shandong provinces.

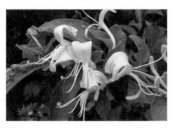

Properties and taste: Cold; sweet

Channels of entry: Lung, heart and stomach

Composition and pharmacology: The high chlorogenic acid and isochlorogenic acid contained in honeysuckle may help strengthen the immune system against infections.

Culinary usage and medical applications:

Clearing away heat and toxins: Honeysuckle treats wind heat-type common colds and expels early-stage infections. It reduces summer-heat and helps heat rash, boils and carbuncles. It also stops bloody diarrhea caused by appendicitis.

How to eat?

1. Raw: Fresh honeysuckle can be eaten as salad.

2. Tea: Drink tea made with dried honeysuckle to reduce boils. Honeysuckle is also a general cooling tea when eating spicy food.

3. Syrup: Available in Chinese pharmacies, the syrup is used to cool children with summer-heat, and prevent and treat skin rash.

They should drink 10–20ml, 3 times daily.

4. Decoction: A honeysuckle and licorice decoction is good for breast infection, especially mastitis due to breast feeding.

Contraindication:

People with weak and cold constitutions, especially in the stomach, should avoid honeysuckle. Those with muscle swelling, skin ulcer or rash (weak qi type) are prohibited from taking it.

Jujube (Chinese Date) 大枣

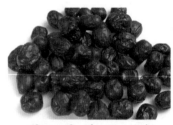

Scientific name and origin: Jujubes are mature fruits of Rhamnaceae. Latin name: *Ziziphus jujuba* Mill. It mainly comes from the Hebei, Henan and Shandong provinces of China.

Properties and taste: Neutral to warm; sweet

Channels of entry: Spleen, stomach and heart

Composition and pharmacology: Zizyphus saponin I, II and III, jujuboside B, stepharine, glucose and fructopyranose are all found in jujubes. Jujubes are a superb functional food, regulating body mechanisms, stopping coughing and reducing phlegm, and restraining nerve centers and calming the mind. Their anti-oxidants protect the liver; anti-cancer properties are also present.

Culinary usage and medical applications:

1. Strengthening the spleen and stomach: Jujubes can treat weak stomach and spleen, as evidenced by shortness of breath, tiredness, aversion to speaking, low appetite, sensations of fullness, distention of stomach and abdomen, and loose bowel movements.

2. Nourishing the blood to tranquilize the mind: Jujubes can ameliorate deficiencies of blood and spleen qi as manifested by insomnia, forgetfulness, palpitations of fear, and poor appetite. They are also useful for liver and heart blood deficiencies, with symptoms that may include irritability, hysteria, lassitude, mood swings, absent-mindedness, light sleeping, confusion,

uncontrollable yawning, laughing or crying, thirst, constipation, and being easily affected by the environment.

3. Easing and reducing the toxicity of other herbs: Jujubes alleviate the side effects of medications. It can decrease the side effects of very strong herbs, and protect the spleen and stomach.

How to eat?

1. Decoction: Chop 10–30g of dry jujubes, boil into a decoction for approximately 20 minutes. They can enrich blood of the heart and strengthen spleen qi.

2. Stewed: Wash and chop 250g chicken and 30 jujubes into bite-sized pieces. Place into a heat-safe bowl along with 5g ground ginger powder and 100ml water. Steam for an hour, adding salt to flavor. This recipe can be good for men with sexual dysfunction or impotence caused by too much sex, often accompanied by dizziness and blurred vision, palpitation, shortness of breath and exhaustion.

3. Soup: Wash 60g jujubes thoroughly; add 180–250ml of water, soak for 15 minutes, then boil for 20 minutes. Eat approximately 20–30 dates and drink 50–80ml of the soup daily for 3 days. This soup is good for weak and cold stomachs, stomach ache and poor appetite.

4. Fresh or dried: Eat 5 to 10 jujubes daily, 2 to 3 hours before bed. If using fresh, be sure to wash thoroughly; cooked dates can also be used. This is good for insomnia.

5. Porridge: Cook 500ml of water, 30g jujubes, 120g rice and 30g dried longan fruit (skin- and pit-removed) together to make porridge. Eat 1 bowl, twice a day. This can nourish the heart, ease the mind, strengthen the spleen, and enrich blood. It is good for people with palpitations, insomnia, amnesia, anemia, spleen weakness with diarrhea, edema, spontaneous perspiration, and night sweats, characteristics of both qi and blood deficiency.

6. Paste: Stew jujubes for about an hour. Remove the skin and pit, and pound into paste adding sugar to taste. This can be used instead of butter or jam on toast or accompanying any other food.

Contraindication:

Jujubes are not suitable for people with phlegm accumulation or poor appetite caused by indigestion.

Kelp 海带

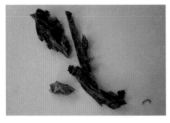

Scientific name and origin: Kelp is a thallus of the Laminariaceae family, with the Latin name of *Laminaria japonica* Aresch; or Alariaceae family, with the Latin name of *Ecklonia kurome* Okam. In China, kelp primarily comes from Shandong, Liaoning and Zhejiang provinces.

Properties and taste: Cold; slightly salty

Channels of entry: Kidney and liver

Composition and pharmacology: Kelp is high in iodine, and is a supplement for iodine deficiency. It also contains pentosan, grass wrack, galacturonic acid, tannin and vitamin B2. Kelp is thought to lower blood pressure and prevent platelet blockages. It also strengthens the heart and reduces lipid levels. Kelp can reduce susceptibility to radiation and some cancers. It counters the effects of vitamin B deficiency with its high B2 levels.

Culinary usage and medical applications:

1. Softening: Kelp works to reduce phlegm and soften or even eliminate lumps and knots. It helps prevent thyroid or lymphatic system problems.

2. Diuretic: Kelp is a diuretic, and reduces swelling.

How to eat?

1. Raw: Eat as starter with garlic or chili.

2. Soup: Kelp can be made into soup with radishes. To counter heart palpitations accompanied by lower body water retention and productive cough, try the following recipe: Soak 30g Job's tears (pearl barley) for about 1 hour. Soak 30g sliced kelp for about 10 minutes, then wash. Add 2 cups water, boil together into soup for 40 minutes, adding pepper to taste.

3. Rehydrated: Kelp can also be served rehydrated, cold, with garlic, sesame seeds, and vinegar or chilies, being sure to avoid salt.

4. Stewed: Mixed with meat, such as pork, kelp can be made into stew; noodles can be added.

5. Stir-fried: To prevent or reduce high blood pressure and tightness in the chest, use the following recipe: Soak 15g sliced kelp and wash as above. Stir-fry with 10g water chestnuts (drained) and 15g sweet corn, or make into a soup.

Contraindication:
Someone who is very weak and extremely susceptible to cold should not eat kelp because of its cold properties.

Do not eat with licorice root.

Kumquat 金橘

Scientific name and origin: Kumquat are mature fruits of the Rutaceae family. Latin name: *Fortunella margarita* (Lour.) Swingle, *F.crassifolid Swingle* and *F.japonica* (Thunb.) Swingle. Within China, they mainly grow in Zhejiang, Fujian, Guangzhou and Anhui provinces.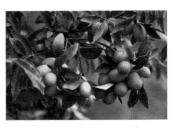

Properties and taste: Warm; sweet, slightly acid and spicy

Channels of entry: Liver, spleen and stomach

Composition and pharmacology: Kumquats contain coniferin and syringin; this composition will serve to raise blood pressure. They also contain citrusin B.C.D and 6, 8-di-C-glucosylapigenin, which can reduce blood pressure. Due to these dual properties, they can be used for diphasic blood pressure regulation.

Culinary usage and medical applications:
1. Moving qi and dispelling phlegm: Kumquats facilitate movement of qi, smooth qi stagnation, and resolve phlegm and productive cough.

2. Treating hangover: Kumquats prevent and treat hangovers after drinking, as accompanied by thirst, chest fullness, and bloating of stomach and abdomen.

3. Regulating digestion: They can also treat poor appetite and pain in the stomach. 9–12g of honey-soaked kumquat can treat

stomach acid and lack of appetite.

How to eat?

1. Fresh: 15–30g, as juice, tea or fruit snack.

2. Preserved with honey: Slice 12g of honey-soaked kumquats, put into a cup, then pour 100ml of boiled water and soak for 10 minutes. Eat the kumquat pieces, and drink the liquid to stop thirst and reduce stomach distention. It can also assist in weight loss. Clinical studies show that using this recipe, 3 times daily for three days, is extremely effective in treating post-surgery abdominal distention.

Contraindication:

People who have dry and hot constitutions should not consume too much.

Lemon 柠檬

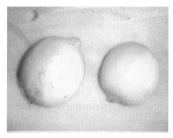

Scientific name and origin: Lemons are fruits of the Rutaceae family. Latin name: *Citrus limonia* Osbeck or *C.limon* (L.) burm.f. *Citrus limonia* mainly grows in Western Asia and southern areas of China. *C.limon* (L.) mainly grows in Guangdong, Guangxi and Guizhou provinces in China.

Properties and taste: Cool; acid and sweet

Channels of entry: Stomach and lung

Composition and pharmacology: Substances called limonoids, found in lemons, may fight various cancers, including mouth, skin, lung, breast, stomach and colon cancer. The vitamin C content of lemons (and limes) can boost and strengthen the immune system, and guard against conditions such as bronchitis, the common cold, ear infection, fever, flu and hives. Lemon also contains hesperidin, β -sitosterol and diosmin. It is an anti-bacterial and anti-viral as well as having anti-inflammation and anti-oxidant properties (lemons harvested in July have the most effective function), and can stop bleeding. Lemon juice with seeds contains limonin, which has sperm-killing results.

Culinary usage and medical applications:

1. Producing fluid and arresting thirst: Lemon increases production of body fluid, helping to relieve dry skin and constipation.

2. Clearing summer-heat: Lemon cools summer-heat with thirst and irritability, and is commonly used for making iced tea. It also reduces stomach heat and thirst.

3. Regulating digestive qi: Lemon harmonizes the stomach and can calm a fetus. It helps treat dry cough, irritability, thirst and poor appetite, as well as nausea, stomach and abdomen distention, belching and hiccups, and morning sickness. Clinical reports show that lemon can have beneficial effects after surgery. Sniffing lemon fragrance a few times after gynecological operations can prevent and treat nausea and vomiting.

4. Resolving phlegm and arresting cough: Lemon also helps productive cough and phlegm heat cough.

5. Treating swelling. It can be used externally against mastitis.

6. Regulating blood circulation: It works again stagnation, thus improving the healthy appearance of facial and body skin.

How to eat?

1. Raw or juiced

2. Fruit wine: Slice 4 lemons, remove seeds, then add one sliced apple; soak in a bottle of rice wine for three months. Drink 20ml per day until the bottle is finished.

3. Tea: Slice 1–2 lemons (fresh or dried) and use for tea.

4. Decoction: Lemon mixed with other herbs can be cooked as a decocted drink.

5. External use: For mastitis, soak cotton with the juice of one lemon, apply to breast, then cover with plastic wrap.

Licorice Root 甘草

Scientific name and origin: Licorice is the root and stem of *Glycyrrhiza uralensis* Fisch., or *G.inflata* Bat. and *G.glabra* L.

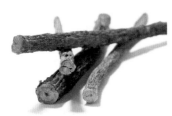

Licorice belongs to Leguminosae. In China, it is mainly produced in Inner Mongolia, Xinjiang and Gansu provinces.

Properties and taste: Neutral; sweet

Channels of entry: Heart, lung, spleen and stomach

Composition and pharmacology: Licorice root contains glycyrrhizic acid, glycyrrhizin, glycyrrhetinic acid, monoamine, various kinds of amino acid and sweet elements. Licorice regulates the immune system, protects the liver, reduces blood fat and serves as an anti-oxidant. It also has anti-inflammation, anti-ulcer, anti-virus, anti-tumor and anti-arrhythmia properties. Licorice stimulates secretion of the pancreas, adjusts movements of the stomach and bowels, stops coughing and disperses phlegm.

Culinary usage and medical applications:

1. Supporting the heart and spleen: Licorice can be used in cases of reduced heart qi, with symptoms of heart pain and pale face, breathlessness after exercise, palpitations, light coating on the tongue and weak pulse. It is also applicable to liver problems with feelings of irritability and anger that is quick and uncontrollable. It can remedy spleen and stomach weakness, manifested by a full feeling in the stomach and constipation, accompanied by breathlessness, weak voice and fatigue.

2. Moisturizing the lung and stopping cough: Licorice can treat coughing, and is applicable to cold, hot and weak situations. Coughing caused by cold can be marked by constant coughing, breathlessness, white and watery phlegm, and feeling cold. If the coughing type is hot, it is accompanied by feeling hot, breathlessness, yellow and thick phlegm, and high fever. If the lung is dry and weak, the coughing may be silent, there is less phlegm and the sticky mucus is difficult to expel.

3. Relieving and stopping aches: Applicable to weak lung and cold stomach conditions, licorice can treat symptoms such as serious abdominal ache and a frozen or numb feeling in the limbs during to lack of blood circulation.

4. Detoxifying: Licorice decreases the toxicity and side effects

caused by other medicines, and protects the spleen and stomach.

How to eat?

1. Candy: Natural candy made from licorice is good for smoothing skin and improving mood. It is also generally refreshing.

2. Powder: Dry and pound 50g licorice into powder, and mix with honey to make pills (the size of small beans). These are useful against coughing in children.

3. Porridge: Place 3g roses, 6g honeysuckle and 6g licorice into water and boil. Then add 50g brown rice, and cook together as a porridge (congee). Add 1 tsp of honey before eating. This recipe is used for clearing phlegm and regulating the stomach. It also dispels heart heat and brightens the eyes, as well as prevents diarrhea.

4. Tea: Soak 10g of raw licorice in boiling water for 10 minutes, then drink as tea to cure sore throat.

Contraindication:

Not suitable to take with marine algae, Peking euphorbia root, lilac daphne flower bud and Euphorbia kansui.

Licorice must not be used in cases of edema. If one takes a large quantity of raw licorice for too long, water retention, rising blood pressure, headache and other side effects will appear.

Lily Bulb 百合

Scientific name and origin: Lily bulbs are the bulbs of *Lilium brownii F.E. Brown var. Viridulium* Baker and *L. Pumilum* DC. Lily bulbs belong to Liliaceae. They are produced in many regions of China, including Hunan and Zhejiang provinces.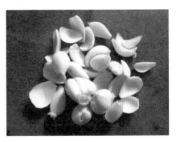

Properties and taste: Slightly cold; sweet and slightly bitter

Channels of entry: Lung and heart

Composition and pharmacology: Lily bulb is full of amylum and proteins. It can improve the immune system, protect membranes in the stomach, stop coughing, drive away phlegm, stop asthma, improve sleep quality, fight fatigue and raise white blood cell counts.

Culinary usage and medical applications:

1. Nourishing lung yin: Lily bulb treats lung yin weak, marked by dry or hoarse cough, and bloody mucus. It also treats afternoon fever; high- or low-grade temperature; heat in the palms, chest and feet; thin and rapid pulse; and a red tongue.

2. Clearing away heart heat to calm: Lily bulb can relax the nerves and hysteria, and relieve some secondary illnesses that develop after certain infectious diseases, where symptoms include low grade fever, dizziness, anger, poor sleep and malaise.

3. Replenishing yin and removing heat of the lung and stomach: Lily bulb can nourish body fluid of the lung and stomach, while removing heat from these organs. It treats "empty heat," as evidenced by a stomach that is painful, upset and noisy; hunger with no desire to eat; dry mouth and throat; and dry stool.

How to eat?

1. Soup: Boil 500ml water, then add 30g of mung beans; bring to a boil again and stew 10 minutes. Then add 60g of lily bulb and stew for another half an hour. Add 3 tsp of honey before serving. This soup can expel summer-heat and toxins while increasing body fluid to quench thirst.

2. Steamed: Wash 60g of fresh lily bulbs thoroughly, then dry. Place lily bulbs and 30g of honey into heat-safe cup and steam for an hour until they become soft. This can help stop coughing in the elderly and children.

3. Juice: Run 100g of lily bulbs through a juicer and then mix with 20ml of warm water. Drink this for coughing with blood.

4. Porridge: Make a simple porridge using 50g of lily bulbs and 100g glutinous rice. Eat this regularly to prevent asthma and cough, and to strengthen weak lung and spleen qi.

5. Stir-fried: Stir-fry with celery or black fungus for 3 minutes to help regulate lung and liver yin, qi or blood.

Contraindication:

In the case of "cold coughing" and "cold stomach," as described in the Licorice section above, combined with diarrhea, lily bulbs must not be eaten.

Longan Fruit (Dragon Eyes) 龙眼肉

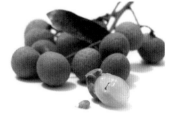

Scientific name and origin: Longan fruits are from the Sapindaceae. Latin name: *Euphoria longan* (Lour.) Steud. In China, they are mainly grown in Guangdong, Fujian and Taiwan.

Properties and taste: Warm; sweet

Channels of entry: Heart and spleen

Composition and pharmacology:

Longan fruit is full of vitamins A, B, and C, glucose and sucrose. It is a functional food that supports weight gain, improves the immune system, and has anti-bacterial, anti-cancer and anti-hormone functions.

Culinary usage and medical applications:

1. Nourishing the heart and invigorating the spleen: Longan fruit strengthens weak heart blood and spleen qi, characterized by yellow face, dizziness, shortness of breath, and weariness.

2. Nourishing blood to calm the mind: The longan fruit can stimulate production of blood and improve mood. It works against anxiousness and preoccupation that affects the heart and spleen, including such symptoms as palpitation, insomnia, forgetfulness and poor appetite.

How to eat?

1. Fresh: 15–30g, as fruit or fruit juice.

2. Stewed: In water, slowly stew 10 to 15g of longan fruit (but for large dosages, no more than 60g), along with other sliced Chinese herbs.

3. Porridge: Remove the skin and pit of 10g of longan fruit, and put in a pot with 100g of rice (washed thoroughly) and 5 pitted jujubes (Chinese dates), along with sugar to taste. Add adequate water and boil into a porridge. Eat once per day to relieve palpitations caused by heart blood deficiency.

4. Tea: Wash 10g of longan fruit, add to boiling water along with 3g of crystal sugar. Let sit for a while and then drink. This drink can be used for treating insomnia, palpitations and excessive dreams, symptoms that demonstrate the need to strengthen the

heart and spleen, and to nourish qi and blood.

5. Jelly: Using low heat, boil 1000g of mulberries, 500g of longan fruit, and sufficient water into an herb jelly. Take twice per day, 10g each time. This jelly benefits the liver and spleen, and nourishes blood, bringing shine to the eyes.

6. Steamed: Using 20ml water and 50g dried longan fruit, steam for 20 minutes. Eat 10g per day, continuing for 5 days, to treat blood deficiency.

Contraindication:

People who have blockages in their middle digestive system caused by dampness or water retention should be wary of longan fruit.

Similarly, people who have too much heat of heart or lung should take with caution.

Loquat Fruit and Leaf 枇杷 枇杷叶

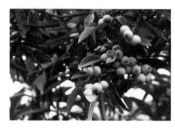

Scientific name and origin: Loquats are fruits of Rosaceae. Latin name: *Eriobotrya japonica* (Thunb.) Lindl. Loquat is originally from the southeastern part of Sichuan province in China. Later it was introduced to Japan, India and the Mediterranean area.

Properties and taste: Cool; sweet and sour (fruit). Cool; bitter (leaf)

Channels of entry: Lung and spleen

Composition and pharmacology: Loquat is low in saturated fat and sodium, and is high in vitamin A, dietary fiber, potassium and manganese. Fresh loquat leaves contain nerolidol, farnesol, amygdalin and malic acid.

Culinary usage and medical applications:

1. Cooling lung heat and stopping cough: Loquat nourishes the respiratory system and quenches thirst. The loquat is comparable with its distant relative, the apple, in many respects, with a high

sugar, acid and pectin content. Besides being eaten fresh, loquats are often served poached in light syrup. Loquat leaf extract, which comprises the leaves combined with other ingredients, acts as an expectorant and soothes dry cough and plum throat.

2. Normalizing the stomach by guiding qi downward: Loquat soothes the digestive system, and acts against hiccupping and vomiting.

How to eat?

1. Fresh: Loquat fruit can be eaten fresh (60–100g) or mixed with other fruits in fruit salads or fruit cups.

2. Pies: Slightly immature fruits are best for making pies or tarts.

3. Jam: The fruits are also commonly used to make jam, jelly and chutney, which can be put on bread or steamed bread.

4. Syrup: Loquat syrup is used in TCM for soothing the throat like a cough drop.

5. Paste: To make loquat paste, use both fruits and leaves combined with other ingredients; this is called *pipagao* (loquat leaf extract). Mix some paste with 10ml warm water and drink or eat as a cough drop.

6. Wine: Loquat can also be made into a light fruit wine, then drink 25ml with meal.

Contraindication:

It is recommended that you do not eat more than 200g of fresh loquat in a single serving as it may induce abdominal fullness, bloating or soft bowel movements.

Loquat syrup should not be taken when cough is accompanied by vomiting.

Lotus Seed, Leaf, Plumule and Root

莲子 荷叶 莲子心 藕

Scientific name and origin: Lotuses are from Nymphaeaceae, with the Latin name of *Nelumbo nucifera* Gaertn. Lotus primarily

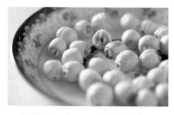

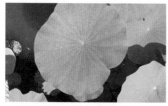

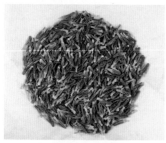

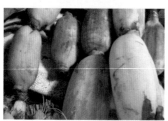

grows in the swamps and lakes of Hunan, Fujian, Jiangsu, Zhejiang and other southern provinces in China. Chinese medicine uses the root, leaf and flower as well as the plumule (shoot). Under the right conditions, lotus seeds can keep reproducing for over one thousand years.

Properties and taste: Neutral; sweet, astringent (seeds). Neutral; bitter, astringent (leaf). Cold; bitter (plumule)

Channels of entry: Spleen, kidney and heart (seeds); heart, liver and spleen (leaf); heart and kidney (plumule)

Composition and pharmacology: Lotus seeds contain β -sitosterol, raffinose, proteins, calcium, iron and phosphorus. They can improve immunity and control blood sugar levels. The plumule contains liensinine and neferine, which can lower blood pressure and act as an anti-arrhythmia agent.

Culinary usage and medical applications:

Seeds

Preserving kidney essence: The seeds invigorate the spleen and stomach, astringe the intestines, relieve diarrhea, arrest seminal emission and treat ongoing diarrhea. They also prevent spontaneous emission, involuntary urination, leukorrhea, dysfunctional uterine bleeding, insomnia, nervousness and jumpiness.

Leaves

Reducing summer-heat: The leaves can help summer dizziness with fullness of chest and abdomen, invigorate the spleen to raise qi to the sense organs, and treat indigestion.

Plumule

Reducing liver heat and calming the mind: The plumule can be used as an herb to nourish the heart, harmonize the heart and kidney, treat irritability and insomnia as accompanied by itchy, red eyes and dizziness.

Root

Regulating blood stasis and stopping bleeding.

How to eat?

1. Raw: Lotus seeds can be eaten fresh in summer.

2. Dried: Lotus seeds, leaves and plumules are most commonly found in dried form. Lotus seeds can be made into desserts or boiled into soup.

3. Stir-fried: Lotus root is a good addition to stir-fried dishes.

4. Tea: Lotus plumule (2g) can be drunk as tea with honey for calm sleep; lotus leaves (3–6g) can be drunk as tea to prevent high blood fat and constipation.

5. Decoction: Using 10g cooked lotus root, 8 jujubes and 1 cup water, make a decoction. Drink the liquid and eat the jujubes to stop vomiting blood, bloody stool and menstrual bleeding.

6. Porridge: Lotus seeds can be made into porridge when combined with millet and jujubes; this porridge helps to strengthen the digestive system and brings sound sleep.

7. Powder: Powdered lotus seeds are sometimes made into Chinese Moon Cake filling and some other snacks. Grind lotus seeds and oyster shells together into powder and mix with rice soup to treat spontaneous sweating.

8. Capsule or extract: Take 3–6g dried lotus leaf powder (as capsule or extract) in the summer to help reduce symptoms caused by summer-heat.

Contraindication:

Do not eat lotus seeds when suffering abdominal distention and constipation.

Avoid plumule or leaf tea if you have a weak stomach and are averse to cold drinks.

Lychee 荔枝

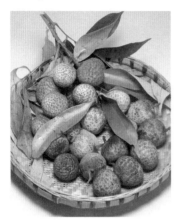

Scientific name and origin: Lychees are fruits of Sapindaceae (Soapberry family). Latin name: *Litchi chinensis* Sonn. The earliest record of lychees is from the Song dynasty (960–1279) in China. They mainly grow in the southeast, east and southwest provinces of China.

Properties and taste: Warm; sweet, acid

Channels of entry: Liver and spleen

Composition and pharmacology: Lychee contains glucose, proteins, vitamin C and lemon acid.

Culinary usage and medical applications:

1. Producing bodily fluid and nourishing blood: Lychee fruit quenches thirst, relieves cough, calms the mind, and relieves palpitations. It clears up acne, pustules, canker sores and mouth ulcers, and moisturizes face skin. Due to this function of nourishment, it is the "queen of fruits" for skin beauty.

2. Strengthening the spleen and liver: Through these qualities, lychee can treat stomach yin weakness marked by irritability, thirst, nausea and stomach ache. It also treats spleen deficiency, which otherwise could lead to lack of appetite or diarrhea.

3. Dispelling swelling and pain: Lychee seeds and plant bark can relieve pain and knots, tranquilize cough, and prevent and treat hernia.

How to eat?

1. Raw: Eating 50g of fresh lychees can treat dry skin with wrinkles, thirst, toothache or soreness, and a swollen throat. For chronic diarrhea, eat 14 lychees and 10 jujubes for 3 days.

2. Dried fruit: For women with heavy and long menstruation, accompanied by tiredness and anemia, use 30g dried lychees to make soup for 5 days. To improve qi and blood deficiency due to giving birth or senile weakness, use 20g dried lychees and 100g

oats to make porridge for breakfast, and eat for a week.

3. Decoction: The following decoction can ease hernias with cold stomach, fullness, distention and abdominal pain: Boil 30–60g of fresh lychee root to make a decoction. Add brown sugar to taste and drink for a course of 5 days.

4. Wine: Lychees are also made into fruit wine or potent liquor, which can warm the body and aid sleep. The following recipe can help impotence, premature ejaculation, mental and body fatigue, and weakness of the knees or lumbar area: Remove the skin of 500g fresh lychees, soak in 500ml high-percent Chinese distilled liquor for a week. Then drink 20ml twice a day until finished.

Contraindication:

If your body feels hot, dry and weak, with heartburn and constipation, or there is an accumulation of yellow phlegm, you should eat with caution.

Malt 麦芽

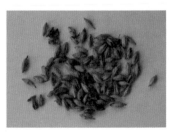

Scientific name and origin: Malt belongs to the Poaceae family; it comes from the dried mature caryopsis sprout of barley. Latin name: *Hordeum vulgare*. L. Malt is produced all over China.

Properties and taste: Neutral; sweet

Channels of entry: Spleen, stomach, liver

Composition and pharmacology: Malt contains hordenine, hordatine A and B, and is high in vitamin B. It contains enzymes that aid in digestion of lactose and starches such as wheat or gluten. It also improves overall digestion and is beneficial to blood sugar and lipid levels.

Culinary usage and medical applications:

1. Aiding digestion: Malt can deal with undigested rice, wheat and potato as well as the associated symptoms of fullness, gas and sour taste. It protects the liver by warding off fungus.

2. Stopping breast milk: Raw malt can help dry up milk when

a mother is ready to stop breast feeding.

3. Treating skin conditions: It is effective against athlete's foot.

How to eat?

1. Flour: Malt flour can be substituted for 50% of the white flour when making bread or pancakes. This alleviates indigestion, poor appetite and distension.

2. Tea: Add cooked malt granules to tea, boiling for 10 minutes; drink twice a day. This tea is good for chronic diarrhea.

3. Powder: Malt powder can be used as a thickener for soups or porridge.

4. Candy: Malt sugar can be eaten as a candy to ease ulcers or for its cooling effects.

5. Decoction: Take 50–100g of raw malt, boil with 2–3 cups of water for 20 minutes, then drink the liquid. Continue for 3 days to stop breast milk.

6. External use: Combine 40g malt and 100ml rubbing alcohol (75%). Let sit for 1 week, then rub on affected area twice a day for 15 days to treat athlete's foot.

Contraindication:

For women who want to continue breast feeding, malt should be avoided.

Moldy malt or malt showing signs of fungus should never be used.

Don't overcook malt.

Marine Algae 海藻

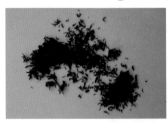

Scientific name and origin: Marine algae are fronds of *Sargassum fusiforme* (Harv.) Setch and *S.pallidum* (Turn.) C. Ag., belonging to the Sargassaceae family. They are found in China as follows: *Sargassum fusiforme* in Shandong and Liaoning provinces, and *S.pallidum* in Fujian, Zhejiang and Guangdong provinces.

Properties and taste: Cold; bitter and salty

Channels of entry: Liver, stomach and kidney

Composition and pharmacology: Marine algae contain a fair amount of iron, which is helpful for preventing and treating anemia and fatigue. They contain unique substances called fucans, which can reduce the body's inflammatory response. They can also help restore sleep. In addition, marine algae contain alginic acid, (SFPP) A, B, C, laminarin and sargassan. Algae can reduce blood pressure, act as a blood thinner and lower blood lipids. They also improve immunity, and act as anti-oxidation and anti-tumor agents.

Culinary usage and medical applications:

1. Dispelling phlegm: Marine algae are noted for the ability to dispel phlegm and soften lumps. Marine algae are used by patients who have an enlarged thyroid or who have lumps on their thyroid; however it is not safe if iodine or thyroxine levels (T3/T4) are elevated. Swollen lymph nodes as a result of common infection can also be treated with marine algae, but not in the case of tuberculosis.

2. Enhancing immunity: From middle age on, if the immune system is weak, warts are more likely to grow, or hernias to develop, in which case marine algae can be used.

3. Improving appearance: Used topically, marine algae can reduce pigmentation, wrinkles and under-eye bags.

4. Controlling weight: Marine algae can treat simple obesity.

5. Cooling internal heat and promoting urination: Algae can cool the blood, reduce hot feelings in early-stage high blood pressure, and soften hardening arteries. Algae can also increase urine to reduce distension.

How to eat?

1. Capsules and powder: These are the most commonly found forms of marine algae. Follow the dosage given on the package. To help treat obesity, eat 6g of marine algae powder, 3 times a day before food, for a month.

2. Decoction: Marine algae also can be boiled with kelp to treat lumps and cysts that grow in between the tendons and below the surface of the skin.

Contraindication:

People who are averse to cold, especially water retention and being stuffed up with white mucus, or who suffer from acute indigestion and bloating, should not consume marine algae.

Do not take marine algae with licorice.

Mint 薄荷

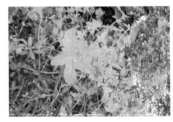

Scientific name and origin: Mint comes from leaves and stems of the Lamiaceae family, with the Latin name of *Mentha haplocalyx* Briq. Mint is mainly grown in Jiangsu province.

Properties and taste: Cool; pungent

Channels of entry: Lung and liver

Composition and pharmacology: Mint contains mint volatile oil, aliphatic acid, mint alcohol and menthol crystals. It induces perspiration, dispels fever, works against spasms and coughing, dispels mucus, functions as an anti-bacterial, and regulates gall bladder to excrete bile.

Culinary usage and medical applications:

1. Expelling wind and heat: Mint prevents and treats flu, sinus, fever, headache from cold, sore throat and stuffy nose. It is useful in the feverish stage of colds and flu, as it promotes perspiration and brings down the body temperature by opening up blood-flow to the skin. Treating the nose with paste, cream or essential oil made from mint helps against stuffy nose.

2. Regulating qi in the liver: Mint treats stagnation of liver qi, indicated by depression, chest and rib fullness and pain, and irregular menstruation.

3. Cooling summer-heat: Mint is an ideal food during the heat and humidity of summer, working against stomach bloating, vomiting, diarrhea and dizziness with heat flush. Mint paste, cream or essential oil can be applied to the head for refreshment.

How to eat?

1. Raw: Fresh mint mingles well with salad.

2. Tea: Mint tea is delicious and beneficial for the digestion, allaying nausea and reducing colic and flatulence in the bowel. It is effective even in conditions as severe as colitis. An infusion should be taken before or after meals to aid digestion, or whenever a pleasant-tasting alternative to ordinary tea is desired.

3. Gum: To refresh mouth or treat toothache.

4. Decoction: To treat chronic skin rash, make a decoction from 15g of mint and 9g of longan fruit. Drink 100ml as a dose, twice a day, for 4 weeks. To refresh the mouth or treat toothache, mix 1g of clove, 1g mint, 2g honeysuckle and 50ml mineral water. Let sit for an hour and use the fluid as a topical refresher, three times per day, continuing for 5 days.

Contraindication:

People with damp and dry constitutions or weakness in blood and body fluids are prohibited from taking mint.

Mulberry Fruit and Leaf 桑椹子 桑叶

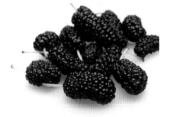

Scientific name and origin: Mulberry fruit and leaf are from the Moraceae family. Latin name: *Morus alba* L. They mainly grow in China's Jiangsu, Zhejiang and Hunan provinces.

Properties and taste: Cold; sweet and acid (fruit). Cold; bitter and sweet (leaf)

Channels of entry: Liver and kidney (fruit); Lung and liver (leaf)

Composition and pharmacology: The total polysaccharides in mulberry leaves help lower blood sugar, boost the immune system, and serve as an anti-bacterial and anti-inflammatory agent. Mulberry fruit also can boost the immune

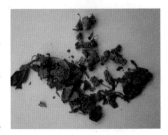

system and increase blood count. Special enzymes in mulberry fruit lower enzymatic activity.

Culinary usage and medical applications:
Fruit
1. Nourishing yin and increasing products of blood: Mulberry fruit prevents and treats dizziness, tinnitus, premature grey hair and weak lower back.

2. Enriching body fluid and moisturizing dryness: The fruit also prevents and treats dry stool and rapid hair loss.

Leaf
1. Expelling wind and heat: Mulberry leaves help at the onset of flu, accompanied by fever, headache, cough and chest pain.

2. Cooling and moisturizing the lung: The leaves help dry mouth and throat, and relieve thirst.

3. Reducing liver heat to treat the eyes: They can also treat red, swelling or painful eyes.

How to eat?
1. Raw: Eat 50–100g of fresh mulberry, nourishing the blood and body fluid.

2. Tea: You can use 3–6g of the dried fruit or leaves to make tea.

3. Powder or extract: Take 3g of mulberry leaf powder to treat excessive sweating. Mix 5g of mulberry leaf powder with 5g of sesame seed powder to treat liver weakness.

4. Decoction: 12g of mulberry fruit mixed with sugar will help infant thirst.

Contraindication:
People who have a cold and weak stomach and digestive system, often experiencing loose stool, should use mulberry with caution.

Mume Fruit (Dried Dark Plum or Chinese Plum) 乌梅

Scientific name and origin: Mume fruit is from the Rosaceae family. Latin name: *Armeniaca mume* Sieb (*Prunus mume* Sieb. et

Zucc.). Mume fruit is made from smoked immature green plums, therefore it is also called dried dark plum. Mume fruit can be found in Zhejiang, Fujian and Yunnan provinces in China.

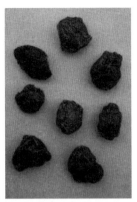

Properties and taste: Neutral; sour and astringent

Channels of entry: Liver, spleen, lung and large intestine

Composition and pharmacology: Mume fruit contains citric acid, malic acid and succinic acid. It promotes gallbladder contraction and secretion. Mume fruit has anti-bacterial and anti-allergic functions.

Culinary usage and medical applications:

1. Astringing the lung to stop coughing: Mume fruit can treat persistent cough due to deficiency of the lung. In these cases, the patients usually cough with little sputum or even without sputum, have shortness of breath and are too tired to talk, typically devolving into chronic respiratory disease.

2. Relieving diarrhea with astringents: Astringent and sour, mume fruit works in the large intestine channel to stop diarrhea. It is one of the common herbs in treating chronic diarrhea due to deficiency of healthy qi.

3. Promoting the production of body fluid: It can promote the secretion of fluid and stop restlessness and thirst, so it is usually applied in treating diabetes with thirst and eagerness to drink due to the deficiency of yin and dryness.

4. Treating warts: It can be used to treat verruca vulgaris or verruca plana.

How to eat?

1. Decoction: Drink 10–12g mume fruit with other herbs in decoction.

2. Dried: Steam with rock sugar and then make into a dry fruit. Eat 3 pieces as a dose, 3 times a day. It can be eaten as a snack to promote fluid production in order to quench thirst as well as

promote digestion.

3. Beverage: Mume fruit juice stops soft stool or diarrhea.

4. External use: Smash rehydrated fruit and spread the juice on affected area to treat warts.

Contraindication:

Those who have acute conditions or excess heat blockage inside the body should avoid mume fruit.

Mung Bean (Green Bean) 绿豆

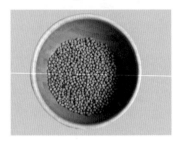

Scientific name and origin: Mung beans are dry seeds of Leguminosae. Latin name: *Vigna radiata* (L.) R. Wilczak (*Phaseolus radiatus* L.). Mung beans are found in most provinces of China.

Properties and taste: Cold; sweet

Channels of entry: Heart, liver and stomach

Composition and pharmacology: Mung beans contain starch, proteins, adipose carbohydrates, lipids, vitamin A, vitamin B-Niacin, phospholipid, calcium, phosphorous, beta carotene and iron. They can reduce high cholesterol, and prevent and treat hardening of the arteries.

Culinary usage and medical applications:

1. Clearing away heat and toxins: Due to their cold nature, mung beans are good at removing toxic heat, treating carbuncles and sores, and soothing flare-ups and pain. Mung beans can be used along with monkshood and croton fruit in detoxification to address restlessness, vomiting and thirst.

2. Removing summer-heat: Again, the cold nature is good for expelling summer-heat, including treating heatstroke, with associated symptoms of sweating, restlessness, thirst, fatigue and occasionally fever or fainting.

3. Inducing diuresis: Mung beans can induce diuresis to

alleviate edema and treat carbuncles and swelling.

How to eat?

1. Raw or fried: Mung bean sprouts can be eaten raw or quickly stir-fried. This method preserves many enzymes and anti-oxidants.

2. Porridge: After soaking 60g mung beans in water for half a day, they can be made into rice porridge. In the summer, this makes a good breakfast or light dinner. This porridge is good for stopping restlessness and thirst; it removes toxic heat and treats edema, especially in the elderly.

3. Flour: After washing the beans, boil them on the stove until they turn to mush. Then add starch and boil until it becomes sticky. Form cakes with the flour and fry on a pan. These cakes can be twisted and unfolded when eating. Soy sauce, vinegar, spicy powder, sesame and garlic are suitable accompaniments.

4. Decoction: Take the following and make into a soup or decoction (as described at the end of this section): Mung beans 50g, azuki beans 50g, black beans 50g, licorice 50g. This recipe can ease hangovers as it flushes alcohol toxins from the body.

Using 60g of mung beans and 60g of dry purslane (if using fresh, 120g), follow the recipe below, and take once or twice a day for 3 days. This can clear heat and detoxify, as well as induce diuresis to alleviate edema.

General recipe: After washing mung beans, boil them (and other ingredients as directed) with 500ml of boiled water, to make a decoction. For the second round of boiling, add 20g of sugar and keep the lid slightly ajar. Boil until the beans are broken but still green, otherwise they lose their effect. This basic decoction is recommended for chronic sore throat, especially during the summer.

Contraindication:

Because of their cold nature, mung beans shouldn't be taken by people who have diarrhea due to cold stomach and deficiency in the spleen.

Mustard Seed 芥子

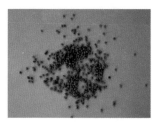

Scientific name and origin: Mustard seeds are from the Cruciferae family. Latin name: *Brassica juncea* (L.) They originated in Europe but now are produced all over China.

Properties and taste: Hot; spicy, slight poisonous

Channels of entry: Stomach and lung

Composition and pharmacology: Mustard seeds mainly contain sinigrin, gluconapin and sinapine.

Culinary usage and medical applications:

1. Aiding the respiratory system: Mustard seeds affect respiration by calming productive cough, resolving phlegm, drying up sputum, relieving fullness in the chest and calming asthma.

2. Regulating the digestive system: They influence the digestive system by warming it, stopping vomiting, and reducing cold abdominal pain.

3. Supporting joints and muscles: The third function of mustard seeds is their ability to counteract arthritis and numbness, dispel swelling and cellulitis, and ease knots and painful muscles and joints. Mustard seed can also treat amenorrhea and deafness.

How to eat?

1. Pickled: Eat pickled with salad.

2. Decoction: Mustards seeds (3–6g) can be used to make a decoction.

3. Powder and pill: Mustard seeds can be powdered and compressed into pill form.

4. External use: To use mustard seeds externally, mix the powder with honey and apply directly on acupuncture points or the affected area for less than 10 minutes.

Contraindication:

Someone suffering from weak lung with chronic cough and dehydration with fever must not take mustard seeds.

Overdosing can cause vomiting and diarrhea.

Mustard oil applied topically is irritating to the skin and can cause burning pain, even blisters, as well as blood congestion. People who have allergies to mustard are advised not to eat mustard or use it externally; people with sensitive skin or a skin ulcer should not use mustard topically.

Nutmeg 肉豆蔻

Scientific name and origin: Nutmeg comes from mature seeds of the Myristacaceae. Latin name: *Myristica fragrans* Houtt. Nutmeg is native to Malaysia and Indonesia, but now limited quantities are also grown in China's Guangdong, Guangxi and Yunnan provinces.

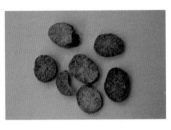

Properties and taste: Warm; spicy and slight bitter

Channels of entry: Spleen, stomach and large intestine

Composition and pharmacology: Nutmeg contains fatty oil, volatile oil and myristicin, which is an anti-inflammatory. (However, in overdose, myristicin and elemicin have shown side effects such as inducing delusions in humans, and liver and brain damage in test animals.) Nutmeg influences the stomach and intestines by relaxing muscle contractions, calms the mind and counteracts tumors.

Culinary usage and medical applications:

1. Warming the internal system: Nutmeg is good for a cold constitution. It warms and regulates the movement of the digestive system to prevent bloating pain, poor appetite and vomiting.

2. Arresting diarrhea: Nutmeg is astringent to the colon thus reducing diarrhea in weak and cold constitutions. In TCM practice, nutmeg is particularly used to treat early morning diarrhea.

How to eat?

1. Cooking with powder: Using 1.5–3g of nutmeg powder is enough. Over dosage can be poisonous.

2. Decoction: Use 3–6g of nutmeg decocted with cloves to

help abdominal pain and diarrhea.

Contraindication:

People who have a damp-heat constitution accompanied by diarrhea should not take nutmeg.

Over dosage (10g of powder) can induce dizziness, coma and death; more than 7g can be poisonous.

Olive 橄欖

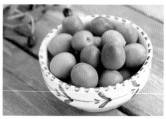

Scientific name and origin: Olives are fruits of Burseraceae, with the Latin name of *Canarium album* (Lour.) Raeusch. They grow in Taiwan, Fujian, Guangdong and Guangxi provinces.

Properties and taste: Neutral; sweet, sour and astringent

Channels of entry: Lung and stomach

Composition and pharmacology: Olives are composed of scoparone, scopoletin and gallic acid. Olive extract can protect against liver damage, and activate the salivary glands to increase secretion, thus aiding digestive function. Olive oil has many beneficial properties. In studies, the exclusive use of olive oil resulted in a 47% reduced risk of coronary heart disease. People with diabetes who consume olive oil may have better insulin sensitivity. Oleic acid, the main monounsaturated fatty acid in olive oil, can reduce the impact of a factor associated with the aggressive growth of breast cancer tumors. Olive oil greatly reduces ulcer size and significantly improves ulcer healing.

Culinary usage and medical applications:

1. Cooling the body, dispelling toxins and enhancing moisture: Olives cool the body, dispel toxins (such as those that cause cold sores), soothe sore throats, and increase production of body fluids to help deal with conditions ranging from cracked lips to dysentery. They can also prevent summer-heat as shown by cough with bloody mucus and swelling. External use of olive oil can prevent

dry cracked skin on hands and feet. Olive oil used to wash hair also has moisturizing benefits. Fresh olive juice (1–2 cups) is useful for relieving buildups of fish and crab poison.

2. Reducing pain: A decoction made from the root of olive trees can treat aches, pains and numbness in the low back, knees and limbs, especially rheumatic arthritis or post-natal arthritis.

3. Acting against cholesterol: Olive oil used in cooking can increase the metabolism of cholesterol, thus preventing high cholesterol.

How to eat?

1. Juice: Fresh olive juice is helpful for sore throat. Take five fresh olives, 450g of fresh radish, and make juice. Drink freshly-prepared juice, continuing for 3 days, for common cold with cough and sore throat.

2. Dried: Dried olives make a good snack between meals.

3. Pickled: Pickled olives can be eaten with salad or as an appetizer.

4. Olive oil: Using olive oil to cook food can help reduce blood cholesterol.

5. Decoction: As mentioned above, decoctions are made both from the olive fruit and other parts of the tree.

Contraindication:

While olives are good for all constitutions, people who are averse to cold, or have a weak stomach or constipation, should take caution.

Oyster Meat and Shell 牡蛎 牡蛎壳

Scientific name and origin: Oysters are from the family Ostreae, with the Latin name: *Ostrea gigas* Thunberg, *Ostrea talienwhanensis* Crosse, or *Ostrea rivularis* Gould. They can be found along the coast of China.

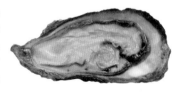

Properties and taste: Neutral; sweet and salty (meat). Slight cold;

salty (shell)

Channels of entry: Lung and heart (meat); Liver, gall bladder and kidney (shell)

Composition and pharmacology: Oyster shells contain various minerals, including calcium, iron, zinc, manganese and chromium, as well as polysaccharose. The minerals tranquilize pain and the mind, and reduce fear and feelings of fainting. Cooked oyster shells can reduce the activity of gastric ulcers. The polysaccharose in oyster shells fights blood lipids and thrombosis, and act as a blood thinner.

Culinary usage and medical applications:

1. Nourishing body yin and blood, quieting the spirit: Oyster calms the mind, and treats irritability, palpitation and insomnia during the summer or in people with a hot constitution. Oyster can prevent and treat hot feelings, feelings of annoyance, malaise, indecision and inability to fall asleep.

2. Softening lumps and reducing swelling: The shells dispel lymph knots, especially those on the neck due to lymph tuberculosis. They can also soften hardened masses.

How to eat?

Meat

1. Raw or cooked: Fresh oysters can be eaten raw or cooked, with methods including frying and boiling.

2. Oyster oil: Oyster oil or sauce is widely available and used in cooking.

Shells

1. Decoction: Make a decoction of 30g cooked, dry oyster shells and drink 50ml, twice a day, for stomach acid regurgitation.

2. Powder: 5g powder of cooked oysters can treat night sweating.

Contraindication:

People with weak digestive systems, diarrhea or heavy vaginal discharge should not eat too much oyster meat.

People with stones (gall bladder, kidney) should be cautious when using oyster shells for medication.

Papaya 番木瓜

Scientific name and origin: Papayas are fruits of the Caricaceae family. Latin name: *Carica papaya* L. Papaya originally grows in South America as well as Guangdong and Taiwan in China.

Properties and taste: Neutral; sweet

Channels of entry: Lung and stomach

Composition and pharmacology: Papaya contains papain and chymopapain A, B and C. The fiber in papaya helps lower cholesterol and reduces the risk of colon cancer by binding to toxins in the

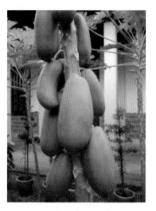

colon and removing them. Special enzymes in papaya reduce inflammation. Papaya also aids digestion, and thus provides relief for condition such as heartburn, irritable bowel syndrome and ulcers. The seeds of papaya impede the fertilization function of males according to animal tests.

Culinary usage and medical applications:

1. Strengthening the spleen and stomach: Papaya works to aids digestion and remove food stagnation. Green papaya promotes lactation in postnatal woman. It treats lack of appetite, stomach ache, poor digestion, and stomach and colon ulcer.

2. Expelling dampness and parasites: Papaya reduces dampness and opens up channels in the body. It helps chronic cough, and reduces numbness and joint pain, for instance stiffness in the neck and shoulder, and low back pain, as well as calf spasm. Green papaya is also used to treat children for tapeworm or roundworm.

3. Treating eczema: Papaya is used externally for infant eczema.

How to eat?

1. Raw: Eating raw papaya (30–60g a day) helps reduce water retention.

2. Steamed: Steam papaya with silver ear to bring moisture to the lung and skin.

For stiffness in neck and shoulder, calf spasm or low back pain, steam one whole fresh papaya (or dried papaya 9–15g) with preserved rice wine for 30 minutes. Divide into two portions. Take one portion every night for 6 days.

3. Juice: Papaya juice combined with milk is a popular beverage in Taiwan.

4. Powder: Make powder from one dried papaya, and take a $^1/_2$ tsp of powder before food to get rid of parasites.

Peach and Peach Kernel 桃 桃仁

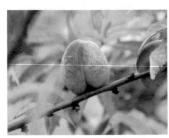

Scientific name and origin: Peaches (hair peach or mountain peach) are fruits of the Rosaceae family. Latin name: *Amygdalus persica* L. or *A. davidiana* (Carr.). In China, *Amygdalus persica* is grown in many places, while *A. davidiana* grows in regions near Hebei and Shanxi provinces. Both fresh peaches and immature green peaches (about the size of a ping pong ball) are used. The inside of the peach pit, called the peach kernel, can also be used after special preparation to neutralize toxins.

Properties and taste: Warm; sweet and sour (fruit). Neutral; sweet and bitter (kernel)

Channels of entry: Lung and large intestine (fruit); Liver, heart and large intestine (kernel)

Composition and pharmacology: The fruit of the peach contains high levels of iron and some protein and fat, as well as soluble fiber, beta carotene and vitamin C. Peaches are composed of organic acids and flavonoids. The kernel contains amygdalin, prunasin, triolein and vitamin B1. It increases blood flow volume and improves micro-circulation, especially in the liver. It has anti-coagulation, anti-thrombosis and anti-inflammatory properties. In addition, it can relieve cough and eliminate phlegm, and can even help digest the protein coating of cancer, allowing for the cancer cell to be eliminated.

Culinary usage and medical applications:

1. Increasing fluids and nourishing blood.

2. Moistening the colon, and moving qi and blood: The peach kernel nourishes the large intestine and colon, strengthens qi and regulates blood circulation.

3. Stopping sweating: Dried immature green peaches can relieve night and spontaneous sweating.

How to eat?

1. Raw: Fresh peaches can prevent dry mouth, and alleviate thirst, constipation and delayed menstruation.

2. Preserved fruit: Eat as a snack or an accompaniment to other food.

3. Decoction and powder: Take dried powder of the kernel to make a decoction. Drink to treat painful or lack of menstruation, abdominal pain after childbirth, cysts in the ovarian or uterus, lung tumor or acute injury.

To regulate high blood pressure, and ease headaches and constipation, boil kernel 10g, cassia seeds 12g and 150ml water for 15 minutes. Drink one glass immediately; take for a maximum of three days.

Contraindication:

Avoid peaches if experiencing diarrhea.

People who bruise easily or are prone to excess blood loss should not eat peach kernel.

Peanut 落花生

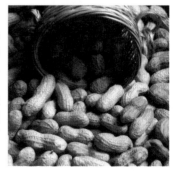

Scientific name and origin: Peanuts are mature seeds of Lequminosae, with the Latin name of *Arachis hypogaea* L. They grow all over China.

Properties and taste: Neutral; sweet (nut). Neutral; sweet, slight bitter and astringent (shell)

Channels of entry: Spleen and lung

Composition and pharmacology: Peanuts contain lecithine, vitamin B1 and the minerals chromium, cobalt, iron and zinc. They slow heartbeat and improve micro-circulation of the blood. The shell contains B-sitosterol and palmitic acid, and has a blood thinning effect.

Culinary usage and medical applications:

1. Moistening the lung, smoothing the bowel: Peanuts moisten lung, resolve phlegm and prevent and treat dry cough. They also moisten the bowel, treating constipation.

2. Strengthening and regulating spleen and stomach qi: Peanuts strengthen spleen qi, promote lactation, regulate the stomach and arrest bleeding. They can be used to treat regurgitation of liquid, lack of breast milk, vaginal bleeding, diarrhea and edema.

3. Stopping bleeding: The shell has a very strong capacity to stop bleeding.

How to eat?

1. Raw: Eating raw peanuts can moisten the lung and eliminate cough.

2. Boiled: Boil unshelled peanuts with salt to taste, drink the liquid, and eat the nuts to nourish the blood and encourage good sleep. These help the digestive system.

Contraindication:

Be careful of allergic reactions.

People with cold and damp constitutions should not eat more than 30g of peanuts a day, and not more than 3 times per week.

Avoid eating peanuts if you have diarrhea.

Pear 梨

Scientific name and origin: Pears are fruits of the Rosaceae family. Latin name: *Pyrus bretschneideri* Rehd., *P.pyrifolia* (Burm.f.) and *P.ussuriensis* Maxim. Pears grow all over China.

Properties and taste: Cool; sweet and acid

Channels of entry: Lung and stomach

Composition and pharmacology: Pears provide copper, a critical part of the superoxide dismutase process, which is an important anti-oxidant defense, and as such, a key player in preventing cell damage. Pears are less likely than many other fruits to cause adverse reaction in infants, which makes them a good choice as a first fruit. The abundance of fiber in 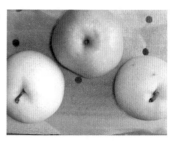 pears helps prevent constipation, promotes regularity, helps reduce cholesterol levels, and aids the removal of toxins from the intestinal tract, which helps prevent colon cancer, diverticular disease, and irritable bowel syndrome.

Culinary usage and medical applications:

1. Promoting body fluid and moistening dryness: Pear increases production of body fluid, quenching thirst and aiding the lung system. Pear strengthens muscle regeneration. It prevents and treats dry mouth and lips, dry and hot cough, sore throat, diabetes, constipation and restlessness.

2. Removing phlegm-heat: Pear also removes phlegm to help cough, and dispels heat and toxins. It can be used to treat thirst, delirium or dysphagia due to acute infection.

How to eat?

1. Raw: Eat a pear, then drink a half-cup of warm water an hour before sleep to prevent constipation.

2. Juice: Mix pear juice, water chestnut juice and asparagus root juice well, and drink fresh to treat hot constitution and thirst.

3. Steamed: Steam together with rock sugar to treat dry cough. Eat once a day for 3 days.

4. Jam: It can also be boiled down into jelly.

5. Dried: People who do not like the fresh fruit may enjoy dried pear.

Contraindication:

People suffering from cold-type cough, or loose stool caused by a weak digestive system, should avoid eating pear.

Pearl Barley (Job's Tears, Coix Seed)

薏苡仁

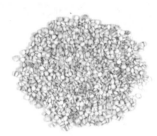

Scientific name and origin: Pearl barley comes from dried and mature seeds of Poaceae. Latin name: *Coix lacryma-jobi* L.var. *ma-yuen* (Romanet.) Stapf. In China, pearl barley is mainly found in Fujian, Hebei and Liaoning provinces.

Properties and taste: Slightly cold; sweet and bland

Channels of entry: Spleen, stomach and lung

Composition and pharmacology: Pearl barley contains fatty oil, coixenolide, coixans A, B and C, protein and vitamin B1. Coix oleic acid contracts the small intestine. Decoctions and alcohol made from pearl barley function against cancer cells and reduce blood sugar. Research shows that pearl barley reduces fever, calms the mind and stops pain.

Culinary usage and medical applications:

1. Eliminating dampness through diuresis: Pearl barley works to reduce dampness and has diuretic properties. It can be used in treating water retention and difficulty in passing urine.

2. Strengthening the spleen: It treats spleen weakness, reducing diarrhea, and also assisting with reducing white and watery vaginal discharge.

3. Eliminating dampness to stop joint pain: Additionally, pearl barley (in combination with other Chinese herbs) is beneficial in the treatment of arthritis and general stiffness and swelling of the joints.

4. Clearing away heat and discharging pus: Barley can treat abscess of the lung and appendicitis. Moreover, it is useful in treating jaundice and warts.

How to eat?

1. Tea: Combine 60g of pearl barley (previously soaked in water for 30 minutes), 25g mung beans or green beans, 10g

hawthorn berries, and 600ml water. Bring to a boil and allow to simmer for 15 minutes. Take off the stove but do not remove the lid for an additional 15 minutes. Then drink the tea and eat the solid ingredients. It is best to drink 100ml to 200ml of the tea daily, 1 to 2 times per day.

To treat urinary tract or bladder infection, and assist with decreasing crystals in the urine, use the following recipe: Boil 50g pearl barley, 125g barley root and 1000ml water for 30 minutes. Allow to cool down, then cook again for 30 minutes. Discard the solids and drink the liquid, twice daily for at least one month.

2. Porridge: Mix 60g of pearl barley (previously soaked for 30 minutes), 100g rice and 1000ml water. Cook in a pressure or rice cooker for 15 minutes. This porridge has anti-cancer properties, and should be consumed 2 to 3 times per week by people who have a family history of cancer.

To prevent children's cold and flu problems, make the following porridge: Mix 30g pearl barley (previously soaked for 1 hour), 30g Dolichos seeds (previously soaked for 30 minutes), 500g rice, and 1.5L of water. Cook for 30 minutes in a pressure or rice cooker. Take twice daily for 5 days.

Contraindication:

Those with spleen deficiency and dry constitution or dry stool should not eat pearl barley.

Do not eat pearl barley when pregnant.

Pepper 胡椒

Scientific name and origin: Peppers are fruits of the Piperaceae family, with the Latin name: *Piper nigrum* L. While pepper is not native to China, it is now found in Henan, Guangdong, Guangxi and Yunnan provinces.

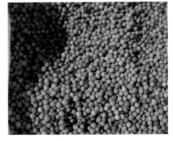

Properties and taste: Hot; pungent
Channels of entry: Stomach, large intestine and liver

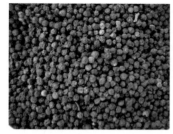

Composition and pharmacology: The alkali in pepper increases blood around the gallbladder, thus aiding bile secretion and acting as an anti-inflammatory.

Culinary usage and medical applications:

1. Warming the middle jiao: By warming the digestive system, pepper dispels cold from the body; prevents and treats stomach ache, vomiting, diarrhea and poor appetite; and thwarts early stage colds from developing in the stomach.

2. Moving the energy down: It stimulates appetite and increases digestion. Pepper moves energy downward in the body, treats epilepsy and watery vomiting, and opens a clogged throat.

3. Clearing away phlegm and toxic materials: Pepper treats white phlegm and food stagnation. It also removes food poisons and treats skin disease caused by poisonous snakes or dog bites. Pepper can be ground into powder for external application.

How to eat?

1. Condiment: Pepper is added as a seasoning in the cooking of various types of foods, such as beef or spaghetti. It also can be used with raw food such as salad.

2. Decoction: Alternatively, it can be made into a medical decoction. To treat stomach ache, poor appetite and cold feelings, grind 10 raw peppers, 3 jujubes and 5 almonds into powder. Drink warm water to help swallow the powder. Continue for 7 days as a course of treatment. Children and those with a weak constitution should take only half the dosage.

Contraindication:

People with the following conditions are prohibited from using pepper as a form of treatment: diabetes, high blood pressure and internal heat.

The following are also advised to avoid it: pregnant women, patients coughing and vomiting blood, and those with a dry-heat constitution. With an eye, ear or nose infection, try to avoid eating pepper.

Persimmon 柿子

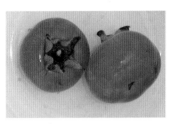

Scientific name and origin: Persimmons are edible fruits of a number of tree species in the genus Diospyros in the ebony wood family (Ebenaceae). In China, they grow in Shandong and Henan provinces.

Properties and taste: Cool; sweet and astringent (fruit). Neutral; bitter and astringent (calyx)

Channels of entry: Heart, lung, large intestine (fruit); stomach (calyx)

Composition and pharmacology: Persimmon is high in glucose, with a balanced protein profile, and has various medicinal and chemical uses. Persimmon contains a number of sugars (sucrose, glucose and fructose), while the immature fruit is composed of tannins, mainly gray glycosides, leucoanthocyanin and citrulline. It is full of iodine, which can help hypothyroid conditions.

Culinary usage and medical applications:

1. Reducing heat, nourishing the lung: Persimmon resolves phlegm and eliminates cough, as well as treating heat-phlegm type cough and chronic bronchitis. It also regenerates body fluid, relieves summer-heat thirst and heals sores in the mouth or mouth ulcers.

2. Invigorating the stomach qi, treating diarrhea with astringents: Persimmon stops bleeding from the stomach, diarrhea and bloody stool as found in those with a hot constitution.

3. Detoxification: Persimmon reduces toxins from drinking too much or allergic reactions to paint.

4. Using the calyx: The calyx that remains attached to the fruit after harvesting also has strong medical functions. It balances qi as associated with symptoms of hiccupping, belching and nausea. Clinical reports also show it can treat hiccups caused by chemotherapy or cerebral hemorrhaging.

How to eat?

Persimmons are eaten fresh or dried, raw or cooked. As persimmons dry, an external layer of white powder, called *shi shuang* (persimmon frost), forms. Shi shuang is not starch; rather it comes from gooey glucose inside that condenses into crystalline form. This also helps preserve the persimmon.

1. Fresh: When eating fresh persimmon, the skin is usually peeled off, and the fruit is cut into quarters or eaten whole like an apple. One way to consume very ripe persimmons, which can have the texture of pudding, is to remove the top with a paring knife and scoop out the flesh with a spoon.

2. Powder: Make a powder from the dried persimmon leaves and then mix with petroleum jelly (such as Vaseline). This can be applied topically to treat skin discolorations such as purpura (3g of leaves, 3 times a day) and chloasma (3 times a day, use 45g to 120g to see an effect). Powdered leaves can be ingested (5–10g of powder, 3 times a day for 9 days) to treat internal organ bleeding, gastric ulcer and bronchiectasis.

3. Dried: Dried persimmon is called *shi bing* (persimmon cake). It is often eaten as a snack or dessert or used for other culinary purposes. Dried persimmon can strengthen weakness and improve dry conditions.

4. Other forms: Persimmon can be found as wine, vinegar, preserved or frozen fruit, or tea.

Contraindication:

Do not eat persimmon with crab, otherwise it can cause stomach cold and ache, or diarrhea.

People who cannot tolerate persimmon, or eat too much, sometimes can get stones in the stomach.

Pine Nut 松子

Scientific name and origin: Pine nuts are seeds of the Pinaceae family. Latin name: *Pinus koraiensis* Sieb.et Zucc. They are grown in northeast areas of China, such as Heilongjiang and Jilin provinces.

Properties and taste: Warm; sweet

Channels of entry: Liver, lung and large intestine

Composition and pharmacology: Pine nuts contain abscisic acid, unsaturated fatty acids like linoleic acid and others. They function as anti-atherosclerosis agents, and dissolve stones in the gall bladder.

Culinary usage and medical applications:

1. Moisturizing dryness: Pine nuts promote the production of body fluid and blood, warm and regulate bowels, and treat dry cough and weak constipation.

2. Nourishing blood: Pine nuts can nourish and moisten blood and body fluids, to prevent and treat loose flesh and fatigue.

3. Expelling wind: Pine nuts help vertigo, arthritis symptoms with no fixed location, and those with yin weakness.

How to eat?

1. Raw: Eat pine nuts as a snack between meals. Or sprinkle on salads with fruits or vegetables.

2. Cooked: Pine nuts have a wonderful flavor when toasted, and can be mixed in cereal or oatmeal for breakfast, or on cakes and dessert.

3. Stir-fried: Pine nuts stir-fried with peas and sweet corn is a common dish in China.

4. Decoction: Pine nuts decocted with semen biota seed can treat dry skin and joint pain.

Contraindication:

People with the following conditions should avoid eating pine nuts: loose stool, spontaneous emission, an accumulation of phlegm, or damp constitution.

Do not eat together with lamb.

Polygonum (Chinese Cornbind) 何首烏

Scientific name and origin: Polygonum is the tuberous root of the Polygonaceae family. Latin name: *Polygonum multiflorum* Thuna. Also know as Chinese cornbind, or knotgrass or knotweed,

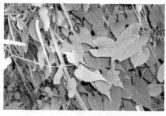

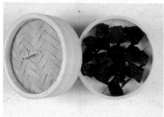

Polygonum is found in most places in China.

Properties and taste: Slightly warm; bitter, sweet and astringent

Channels of entry: Liver, heart and kidney

Composition and pharmacology: Polygonum contains emodin, chrysophanol, physcion and rhein. Polygonum enhances the immune system and has anti-aging properties. It is thought to reduce blood lipids, improve micro-circulation of the blood, and act as an anti-inflammatory.

Culinary usage and medical applications:

1. Nourishing the blood and yin: Polygonum is an effective medical food for strengthening blood and yin, and is one of the "four ancient panaceas" along with Lingzhi mushroom, wild ginseng and Cordyceps sinensis. It can prevent and treat dizziness, light-headedness, palpitations, insomnia and sore or weak lower back and knees. It is noted for its effects on premature grey hair, tinnitus, emission and blurred vision. Long-term consumption of Polygonum improves chances of pregnancy. It is also good for the muscles and bones as it benefits marrow; therefore it aids longevity, is anti-aging and improves vigor.

2. Stimulating bowel movement: Polygonum moistens bowels, preventing and treating constipation of the weak type.

3. Dispelling wind and toxins: Polygonum can be taken to stop itchiness of the skin, and detoxify the body, helping dry skin, rashes, itchy pus and skin lumps. It can also be used externally for skin rashes and scabs.

How to eat?

You can buy Polygonum in raw or cooked form. Raw Polygonum is used to treat constipation, to stop itchiness and to detoxify. Cooked Polygonum is known for nourishing the blood and enhancing production of body fluids.

1. Steamed: Steam and then eat with radish to treat constipation.

2. Tea: Wash 10–15g of Polygonum, then slice or powder for use as tea, adding honey to taste. Drink 3 cups a day to encourage premature grey hair to return to its original color.

3. Soaked in wine: Another treatment for premature grey hair is as follows: Soak 30g cooked Polygonum and 15g angelica in 500ml rice wine. Let sit for 15 days, then drink 30ml twice a day, continuing for 15 days.

4. Powdered or extract: To treat high cholesterol, take 2.5g powder, 3 times a day, continuing for 4 months. Taking 3g of powdered root before bed can encourage sound sleep.

5. Decoction: Decoct 15g Polygonum with 12g Chinese hawthorn berry, take 3 times a week to prevent high cholesterol.

Contraindication:

Those who have "phlegm-dampness" should take with caution.

Do not use iron pots or utensils when preparing Polygonum.

Pomegranate 甜石榴

Scientific name and origin: Pome-
granates are fruits of the Punicaceae family, with the Latin name: *Punica granatum* L. They are native to the Iranian plateau and India, and is now found in China's Jiangsu and Anhui provinces. The most famous ones come from Huaiyuan town in Anhui province.

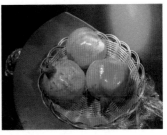

Properties and taste: Warm; sour (fruit); Warm, sour, astringent, mild poison (peel)

Channels of entry: Urinary bladder (fruit); Large intestine (peel)

Composition and pharmacology: Pomegranates have a role in the prevention and treatment of prostate cancer, and appear to act against breast cancer cells. The juice is heart-healthy. It may also help fight erectile dysfunction.

Culinary usage and medical applications:

1. Improving the production of body fluid: Pomegranates stop bleeding, reduce diarrhea, quench thirst and fight dry throat.

2. Eliminating parasites: Pomegranates can be used as pesticide. They treat roundworm inside the body.

3. Using the peel: It is a TCM herb for diarrhea of the cold type.

How to eat?

1. Fresh: Pomegranate can be eaten fresh in different ways. It is great as a juice. For a salad, use a spoon to scrape the pomegranate into a bowl then mix with vegetables and other fruit. You will eat the fruit and seeds together.

2. Alcoholic drink: Put some pulp of pomegranate into champagne for holidays and celebrations.

Contraindication:

Do not eat more than 500g because this may induce phlegm and impair the lung's function.

Potato 马铃薯

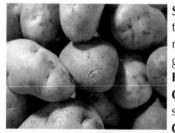

Scientific name and origin: Potatoes are tubers of the Solanaceae family. Latin name: *Solanum tuberosum* L. They grow all over China.

Properties and taste: Neutral; sweet

Channels of entry: Kidney, spleen and stomach

Composition and pharmacology: Potatoes are composed of solanidine, leptinidine, tomatidine, quercetin and tuberonone. They also contain a-solanine and lectin. They are believed to eliminate some carcinogens to prevent cancer. Potatoes have an inhibitory action toward some enzymes, and the patatin in potatoes has anti-oxidant properties, eliminating free radicals. Potatoes can restrain protease activity in the pancreas, and also have a high carbohydrate content, which can lead to obesity when eaten in excess.

Culinary usage and medical applications:

1. Aiding digestion: Potatoes balance the stomach, strengthen qi and body fluid, and help the kidney. Sometimes when people feel lethargic, it is due to weak digestion and failure of the blood to bring new sugar to the muscles; in this case, potatoes can be helpful. Drinking raw potato juice, sometimes combined with honey, can combat duodenum and stomach ulcers and incomplete bowel movements. To prevent or treat constipation, drink raw potato juice on an empty stomach.

2. Dispelling poison and reducing swelling: Drink raw potato juice or use raw potato externally to expel toxins and control swelling. It can also be used topically for eczema and burns.

How to eat?

1. Raw: TCM typically uses raw potatoes for medical use as they are more effective. Don't exceed 100g of raw potatoes per day.

2. Stir-fried: Potato stir-fried with green chili is a dish loved by many children in China.

3. Soup: Potato is a good addition to beef or mixed vegetables soups.

4. Cooked and baked: Western cuisine uses potatoes in favorite recipes among many different cultures.

5. External use: Soak cotton in raw potato juice to use topically on eczema or small burns. For localized eczema, rub on skin 3 times per day continuing for 3 days. For burns, apply once, immediately after the burn occurs.

Contraindication:

Due to the high carbohydrate content, people who have a weak stomach shouldn't eat too many potatoes.

Potatoes that have been fried or processed (such as French fries, chips, etc.) are no longer medically viable and may even be harmful as they could induce allergic reactions.

Do not eat sprouted potatoes or ones that have changed to a brown or purple color. If the potatoes have already sprouted, the chemical compounds have changed, and the effective dosage is different. Potato sprouts are used to reduce spasms and stomach acidity.

Pumpkin and Pumpkin Seed 南瓜 南瓜籽

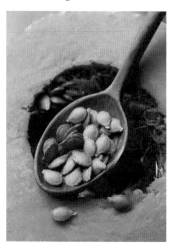

Scientific name and origin: Pumpkin comes from fruit and seeds of the Cucurbitaceae family. Latin name: *Cucurbita moschata* (Duch.ex Lam.) Duch.ex Poir. Pumpkin is found in most places in China.

Properties and taste: Neutral; sweet

Channels of entry: Spleen, stomach and lung (pumpkin); large intestine (seeds)

Composition and pharmacology: The polysaccharides in pumpkin may help reduce blood sugar and lipids. The zinc in pumpkin seeds may help improve bone density. Pumpkin seeds have a high level of phytosterols, which are plant compounds that may reduce cholesterol, boost the immune system, and decrease the risk of some cancers. The high iron content in pumpkin seeds may help if you have anemia or chronic fatigue syndrome.

Culinary usage and medical applications:

1. Strengthening the middle-jiao and aiding qi: Pumpkin treats spleen and stomach deficiency and helps control pulmonary tuberculosis. It is a good staple food to replace rice or bread if suffering from diabetes.

2. Clearing toxins and parasites: Pumpkin clears toxins, eliminates phlegm and purges pus, serving as an anti-inflammatory and analgesic. The seeds treat intestinal parasites.

3. External use: Cooked pumpkin juice can be applied topically to treat rib pain.

How to eat?

1. Boiled: Eat 100g of boiled pumpkin to replace one meal everyday for 5 days to treat early stage diabetes.

2. Steamed: Steam an old pumpkin for an hour, and eat 2tsp before food to help dry cough.

3. Soup: Boil and stew old pumpkin to make soup, especially

good for warming up in winter.

4. Powder: Powder 60g of pumpkin seeds, eat 6g a day for 5 days to treat water retention and diabetes in postpartum women. Children should take 3g twice a day to treat whooping cough.

Contraindication:

People who have dampness and stagnating qi should not eat pumpkin.

Do not cook pumpkin with vinegar, azuki beans or buckwheat, otherwise you will impede the absorption of nutrients.

Radish and Radish Seed   萝卜 莱菔子

Scientific name and origin: These are roots and seeds of the Cruciferae family. Latin name: *Raphanus sativus* L. Usually the large white radish, also known as daikon, is used in TCM, rather than the small, red-skinned radishes often found in salads in the West. It is native to China and grows all over the country. It can be found year round.

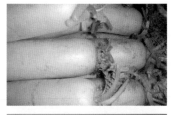
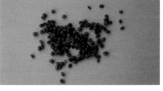

Properties and taste: Neutral to cool; spicy and sweet

Channels of entry: Spleen, stomach, lung and large intestine

Composition and pharmacology: Radishes contain very high levels of phytonutrients called glucosinolates, which are responsible for the secretion of special enzymes that remove cancer-causing substances from the body. Their high fiber content promotes regularity and helps prevent and treat intestinal conditions. The high vitamin C and folate levels may help strengthen the immune system against infections. Radish seeds contain sulforaphane and sinapine. Extract of the seeds can reduce hypertension with a gentle and enduring effect. It increases the rhythmic contraction of the stomach and intestines, and also removes phlegm and stops cough and asthma.

Culinary usage and medical applications:

1. Removing food stagnation: Radish and its seeds aid the function of the digestive system, relieve indigestion and dispel distention.

2. Causing abnormally-ascending qi to descend: Radish and its seeds also regulate qi movement to treat productive cough, wheezing, fullness and pressure in the chest, and lack of appetite.

3. Stopping bleeding: Radish reduces bleeding in cough, vomit and urination.

How to eat?

1. Raw: Radish can be eaten raw with other vegetables.

2. Juice: A mix of radish and hawthorn juices can help infant indigestion. Add 2 tsp to beverage, twice a day for two days; this will treat any breath odor as well as constipation and poor appetite.

3. Soup: Cooked radish can be used in vegetable or meat soups. For example radish and tofu soup is a common everyday dish in China. Five element soup (see recipe in the Beauty section of Chapter 5) can detoxify the body, and help toward achieving ideal weight and preventing tumor growth.

4. Stir-fried: In China, it is popular to eat radish stir-fried with mixed vegetables.

5. Decoction: Radish seed powder and whole seeds decocted with white mustard seeds are used to regulate qi and resolve phlegm.

Contraindication:

People who have qi and yang weakness, or have a dry and weak constitution without indigestion and accumulation of phlegm, should avoid eating too much radish.

Do not combine with ginseng, as radish can reduce the qi-strengthening properties of ginseng.

Rose Bud 玫瑰

Scientific name and origin: Rose buds are flowers of Rosaceae, with the Latin name of *Rosa rugosa* Thunb. Within China, the native region is the north part of China, however they are now found all over China, sourced mostly from Zhejiang and Jiangsu provinces.

Properties and taste: Warm; sweet and bitter

Channels of entry: Liver and spleen

Composition and pharmacology: Rose buds contain rose oxide, a-naginatene, quercetin and cyanin. They increase micro-circulation of the cardiovascular system, and have anti-viral and anti-oxidant effects.

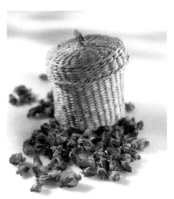

Culinary usage and medical applications:

1. Regulating flow of qi: Rose buds can regulate the body's energy and qi movement. They ease symptoms of PMS, including breast tenderness and distention, as well as irregular menstruation. Rose buds can help break up and dissolve crystallized breast tissue, which would otherwise grow into small lumps. To ease stomach pain and side pain (underneath the ribs), rose buds are often used.

2. Promoting circulation of blood: Rose buds are noted for improving blood circulation especially to the extremities and poorly oxygenated organs or tendons. They work to stabilize water content in blood while balancing the proportions of red and white blood cells, T-cells and platelets to improve overall blood function.

3. Unique harmonizing effects on both qi and blood: Rose bud is noted for its function on both qi and blood; therefore, it is used to bring color back to the face and warm the hands, especially in cold weather. Likewise, tendonitis sufferers, women prone to excessive soreness when wearing high heels, or people who have recently suffered an injury or experience more than mild soreness should drink rose bud tea to enhance both qi and blood circulation to those areas.

4. External use: To counteract stagnation of qi and dissipate blood stasis, use 5g of rose buds in water for a bath or to soak feet for 20 minutes.

How to eat?

When using dried rose buds according to any of the below suggestions, generally 3–6 buds are used.

1. Tea: Dried rose buds are commonly brewed into tea.

2. Desserts: Because of their sweet nature, rose buds can be incorporated into a variety of desserts. To enhance a dessert soup, first soak the dried rose buds allowing them to open up, and then select the best looking ones. Prepare a sweet soup of glutinous rice and sesame balls (which can be bought at Asian markets), adding the rose buds to the boiling water for more flavor and color. Eat the whole soup, including the buds, and drink the liquid. Rose buds (soaked and selected as described above) can also be used to decorate a cake or other dessert.

3. Flour: After grinding the rose buds into powder, the flour can be mixed with baking flour to produce cake, muffins or sweet bread.

4. Wine: Alternatively, the buds can be placed in Chinese distilled liquor, leaving them to infuse, then drinking.

5. Decoction: A decoction using dried rose buds will help symptoms of PMS.

6. Raw: If fresh rose buds are available, and the source is good, this is another option. However the concentration of medicinal properties is not as high in fresh buds, so 10–15 buds (3–10g) should be eaten.

Contraindication:

Rose buds have essentially no contraindications.

Rosemary   迷迭香

Scientific name and origin: Rosemary is whole grass belonging to the Labiatae family, with the Latin name of *Rosmarinus officinalis* L. Rosemary is indigenous to the Mediterranean Sea but now grows in many regions of China.

Properties and taste: Warm; spicy and sweet

Channels of entry: Heart, kidney, liver, lung and spleen

Composition and pharmacology:

Rosemary contains oils, tannins, rosemarinic acid and resins. It helps as a tonic to the liver and circulation, and has a relaxing, restorative effect on the nervous system. Rosemary also acts as an anti-oxidant and restrains auto-immune activity.

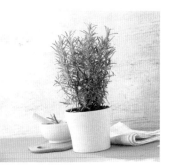

Culinary usage and medical applications:

1. Calming the mind and stopping pain: Rosemary can be used for nervous anxiety, tension and general disability after a long-term nervous or physical illness. It helps relieve tension headaches and may be useful in migraine treatments. Rosemary is believed to strengthen memory and improve heart function.

2. Aiding digestion: People who have a cold stomach, show aversion to cold or dislike raw food can benefit from using rosemary on salad or with vegetables.

3. Opening glands: Rosemary can induce perspiration. The oil can be used externally to help dandruff and poor hair growth. A strong infusion can be applied daily to the scalp, or in the water used for hair-rinsing, to maintain good condition of the hair.

How to eat?

1. Condiment: Rosemary can be used on salad or mixed with vegetables. In western Chinese cooking, rosemary is added to lamb or beef dishes, or else to rice for a hint of flavor. Rosemary is typically sold as a spice, frequently after it has been ground. Fresh rosemary can also be grown at home.

2. Tea: Dried rosemary is sometimes found in tea blends, and likewise you can make your own rosemary tea, adding honey to speed up digestion.

3. Decoction: Make a decoction for hair growth. It should be taken 3 times daily.

Contraindication:

Some people are very strongly allergic to rosemary or to the pollen of the flower, in which case rosemary acts more like a poison.

Safflower and Saffron Crocus 红花 番红花

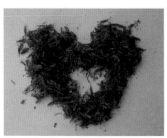

Scientific name and origin: The Latin name of safflower is *Carthamus tinctorius*, of the family Asteraceae; saffron crocus belongs to the family Iridaceae, and its Latin name is *Crocus sativus* L. Its native regions are from southern Europe to Iran. Within China, safflower is commonly grown in Henan, Yunnan, Sichuan, Zhejiang and Jiangsu and is ready for harvesting in the summer. Saffron grown in Tibet and Europe becomes ready in the autumn.

Properties and taste: Warm; spicy (safflower). Neutral; slightly sweet (saffron crocus)

Channels of entry: Heart and liver

Composition and pharmacology: Saffron crocus contains crocin and crocetin. It acts as a blood thinner and increases uterine motion and low blood pressure. It has anti-cancer properties, and can improve memory and learning capacity.

Culinary usage and medical applications:

1. Strengthening the blood, promoting circulation: Both strengthen the blood, but safflower focuses more on circulation while saffron is better at nourishing blood. Through their effect on blood, they can ease pain caused by blood stagnation, such as menstrual or post-partum pain, or lower abdominal pain. Both can address amenorrhea or delayed menstruation, as well as induce labor contractions. If post-partum discharge lasts beyond 15 days, safflower is prescribed to speed up and terminate the process.

2. Treating dry skin and swelling: For dry, scaly, flaky, purplish skin, safflower can help resupply blood to those areas. Safflower is also useful for acute injuries that are accompanied by swelling and bruises.

How to eat?

When using safflower, 6–9g is the typical daily dosage, while for saffron, 0.5–1g is enough. In the winter, when veins have a tendency to close up, half a dosage is sufficient to revitalize blood circulation, especially to the brain.

1. Tea: Dried safflower can be brewed into tea.

2. Spice: Dried saffron crocus is used in cooking.

3. Decoction: Safflower can also be made into a decoction or soaked in wine, and then taken as a drink.

4. Granules: If granules are available, they can be used for tea, mixed into juice or sprinkled on top of salad.

Contraindication:

Pregnant women must not eat safflower, except in the circumstances specified above.

If menstruation is heavy, it is best to avoid it.

If you do not suffer from blood stagnation, there is no reason to take safflower as a medical supplement.

Schisandra Berry　五味子

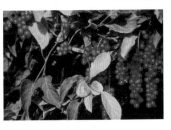

Scientific name and origin: Schisandra berries are mature fruits of the Magnoliaceae family. Latin name: *Schisandra chinesis* (Turcz.) Baill or *Schisandra sphenanthera* Rehd. et Wils. The former is called the northern Schisandra berry and the latter is called the southern Schisandra berry. Schisandra berry is grown in the southern part of the Yangtze River area.

Properties and taste: Warm; sour and astringent

Channels of entry: Lung, heart and kidney

Composition and pharmacology: Schisandra berry contains schizandrin and its derivatives, chlorophyll, sterine, vitamins C and E, resin, tannin and some carbohydrates. It can act on the central nervous system to excite or calm, regulating it to keep balance. The berry is beneficial for the cardiovascular system, prevents kidney and liver disease, reduces stress and regulates breathing.

Culinary usage and medical applications:

1. Supporting the kidney, lung and spleen: The astringent nature of the berry can treat persistent cough caused by weak lung, and sometimes by weak kidneys as well. Clinical symptoms include persistent cough, heavy exhalation with a short inhalation, fatigue and shortness of breath. It can also strengthen the lungs and qi. Schisandra berry is used to suppress sweating in those who sweat spontaneously, have night sweats or severe anxiety-induced sweating. Schisandra berry can support the kidney and strengthen the spleen, especially in people who have diarrhea from too much exposure to cold, are particularly averse to cold, or who have cold limbs.

2. Supplementing qi to promote the production of body fluid: Good for increasing qi and generating bodily fluids, Schisandra berry is used to treat deficiency in those areas. This condition typically manifests as thirst, lassitude, fatigue, shortness of breath and weak pulse; this is particularly common in diabetes patients, who are frequently thirsty and eager to drink.

3. Calming the heart: Schisandra berry can be used to harmonize the kidney and the heart, and calm the mind. In TCM, this condition is thought of as "deficiency in both yin and blood" or a "disharmony of kidney and heart." Symptoms include restlessness, palpitations, insomnia and excessive or jarring dreams.

How to eat?

1. Tea: Crush Schisandra berry, ginseng and longan (skin and pit removed), then add to boiling water for 5 minutes. This tea improves brain function and strengthens spleen qi.

2. Powder: Make a mixed powder from Schisandra berry 35g, tuckahoe 30g, peony 25g and hawthorn fruit 25g. Three times per day, add 3g into drinks or other foods. This mixture is to be used by men for nocturnal emission.

3. Pills: At an herbal or TCM pharmacy, have them make pills using the following powdered ingredients: mulberry 30g, fleece-

flower root 15g, Chinese yam 15g, hawthorn fruit 25g, Schisandra berry 10g and finger citron 10g. Take 3g, 3 times per day for 30 days. For diabetes patients who have a weak kidney, this mixture strengthens the liver and kidneys. It also promotes blood circulation and removes obstructions along the meridians.

4. Porridge: Using 10g of Schisandra berry with 100g rice, make a porridge. The berry enhances liver and kidney function, while the rice protects the stomach and liver. When eaten after drinking alcohol, this porridge can reduce the harmful effects.

5. Decoction: Use Schisandra berry 5g, stem of purple perilla 5g, ginseng 6g and water 300ml, simmering for 30 minutes. Remove and save the liquid, then add another 300ml water to decoct again for another half an hour. Remove the solids, and add 100g sugar to the mixture of the two liquids. This decoction can enhance production of body fluids, reduce thirst, improve deficient conditions, and energize qi; it is particularly useful for patients with cough, stuffy chest, thirst and fatigue.

6. Paste: Use Schisandra berry 250g with honey and sufficient hot water to make a paste. After cooling, the paste can be eaten 1–2 spoonfuls at a time, to treat cough, shortness of breath and weight loss due to weak lung.

Contraindication:

Those who have a persistent bacterial or viral infection, such as the flu or measles, and suffer from fever, should not take Schisandra berries.

Due to the sour and astringent nature of Schisandra berries, people with excessive stomach acid, bloating or water retention should not eat them.

Shiitake Mushroom   香菇

Scientific name and origin: Shiitake mushroom is a dry sporocarp of the Marasmiaceae family. Latin name: *Lentinus edodes* (Berk.) Pegler. Shiitake mushrooms grow in collapsed broad-leaf trees

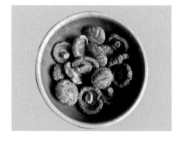

during spring, autumn and winter. They can also be farmed. Shiitake mushrooms are commonly grown in China's Sichuan province, along the central and lower Yangtze River and nearby southern regions, as well as in Japan.

Properties and taste: Neutral; sweet

Channels of entry: Liver and stomach

Composition and pharmacology: The copper in mushrooms may help reduce the symptoms of rheumatoid arthritis and help fight free-radical damage. Shiitakes are composed of unsaturated fats, carbohydrates, crude fiber, calcium, phosphorus, iron and vitamins B1, B2 and D. Shiitakes enhance the immune system, increase lipid fighting activity in cells, promote lymphocyte synthesis, and reduce bodily toxins. They protect the liver by increasing healthy antibodies. Shiitakes have anti-aging and anti-tumor properties, and reduce susceptibility to respiratory infections.

Culinary usage and medical applications:

1. Supporting healthy qi and tonifying deficiency: People known to suffer from a weak constitution, as exemplified by constant feelings of tiredness, aches, lack of energy or lethargy, which may be mistaken as laziness, would benefit from eating shiitakes. Vitamin D deficient people, typically infants and children, who often spontaneously cry at night, suffer from delayed development, or are susceptible to viruses or colds, should consider shiitakes for extra vitamin D.

2. Counteracting fluid retention and toxins: Eaten for five days, 9g daily of shiitakes are useful for people who have fluid retention in the joints (more common in summer). People who suffer from recurring bouts of hives can eat 9–12g of shiitakes per day to reduce frequency and inflammation. To counter the toxic effects of poisonous mushrooms, and to reduce susceptibility to cancer, shiitakes are an effective detoxifying agent. Shiitake mushrooms assist with food poisoning and tumor treatment.

3. Expelling wind: Shiitakes help reduce skin itching and urticaria.

How to eat?

1. Soup: Shiitakes can be added to stews or soups with chicken or other types of meat.

2. Stir-fried: Sliced shiitakes are good in stir-fries.

3. Filling: Shiitakes can be made into filling for dumplings, spring rolls, ravioli or meat pies.

4. Sauce: Mushroom sauce for meats or pasta can be made of shiitakes.

Contraindication:

If the stomach is bloated and retaining water, try to avoid shiitakes.

Shiitakes, when combined with certain types of alcohol, may produce allergic reactions in some people.

Sichuan Pepper (Szechuan Peppercorns)

四川花椒

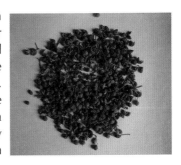

Scientific name and origin: Sichuan pepper (also known as flower pepper and Szechuan peppercorns) is dried fruit of Rutaceae, with the Latin name of *Zanthoxylum bungeanum* Maxim. Typically the dried mature peel of the plant is used. Most places in China grow this pepper, but the best quality is known to come from Sichuan province.

Properties and taste: Warm to hot; spicy

Channels of entry: Spleen, stomach and kidney

Composition and pharmacology: Sichuan pepper contains alkaloid and volatile oil. It is an anti-inflammatory as well as a tranquilizer for pain. It also gives off volatile oils that kill fungus and dust mites.

165

Culinary usage and medical applications:

1. Warming the middle jiao, dispersing cold: Special pharmaceutical functions of Sichuan pepper can treat stomach ulcers. Depending on the dosage, the pepper can regulate wave-like motion in the small intestine: small amounts increase motion, while large amounts reduce too much motion.

2. Improving appetite: People who live in humid areas should consume Sichuan pepper daily to help lack of appetite. It also dispels stagnation of food.

3. Expelling dampness, reducing pain: This pepper can stop abdominal pain accompanied by vomiting and diarrhea. It stops feelings of cold in the joints as well as swelling and pain.

4. Killing parasites and bugs: Sichuan pepper is also known as a killer of intestinal parasites and candida. It gives off volatile oils that kill fungus, dust mites and other bugs. Therefore it is often placed in closets to keep bugs from eating clothing or added to rice bags to discourage infestation.

How to eat?

1. Condiment: Sichuan pepper is typically used to flavor red meats, and in Sichuan cooking, it is even added to vegetables. Many Chinese dishes call for this pepper.

2. Powder: It helps hernia discomfort.

3. Sauce or oil: These can be used to flavor food.

4. Decoction: It can be mixed with other herbs for various decoctions. To kill intestinal parasites, boil 20ml vinegar, 10g Sichuan pepper, 15ml water and sugar (if desired) for 10 minutes. Drink on an empty stomach.

5. External use: Crush 25g Sichuan pepper and 100g garlic until muddled. Rub the mixture directly on skin once to twice daily for two days to kill chronic fungus.

Contraindication:

Pregnant women are advised not to eat Sichuan pepper.

As with chili, people who have a hot and dry constitution should not eat too much.

In cases of constipation, do not eat Sichuan pepper.

Silver Ear (White Fungus)   银耳

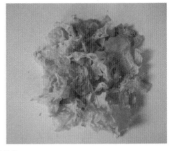

Scientific name and origin: Silver ear is a dry sporocarp of the Tremellaceae family. Latin name: *Tremella fuciformis* Berkeley. Silver ear is commonly grown in China's Sichuan, Fujian, Jiangsu, Zhejiang, Anhui and other nearby provinces.

Properties and taste: Neutral; sweet and bland

Channels of entry: Lung, stomach and kidney

Composition and pharmacology: Silver ear mainly contains tremella polysaccharide, protein, fat, crude fiber, inorganic salt, vitamin B, enzymes and amino acids. It strengthens the immune system, aids protein synthesis and helps the body generate new blood. Silver ear is thought to counter aging and fatigue as well as the effects of radiation. It can reduce lipids in the blood, moderate blood sugar, prevent tumors and ulcers, and act as an anti-inflammatory.

Culinary usage and medical applications:

1. Nourishing yin and promoting body fluid: Silver ear helps weak constitutions after illness, shortness of breath and lack of energy. Those who have low blood pressure or have hearing difficulties (often caused by changes in air pressure on airplanes), should use silver ear with lily bulb.

2. Moistening the lung and strengthening the stomach: Silver ear can strengthen lung qi, indicated by weak, chronic or dry cough, and thick discolored mucus, often accompanied by chest pain or tightness. It is noted for its ability to nourish fluids in the digestive tract, reduce dry mouth and constipation, quench thirst, and reduce both stomach and mouth ulcers.

How to eat?

1. Porridge: Silver ear can be eaten in many of the same ways as wood ear (see Wood Ear section for details) but it is also popular in rice porridge, such as Eight Treasures Porridge.

2. Dessert: It can be incorporated into sweet desserts; silver ear steamed with papaya is a very tasty and popular dessert.

3. Decoction: Silver ear decocted with astragalus root can raise the white blood cell count.

Contraindication:

People with a cough (particularly a productive cough with thick yellow or green phlegm), liquid sputum or aversion to cold, should use with caution.

Soybean, Tofu and Soymilk 黄大豆豆腐豆浆

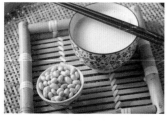

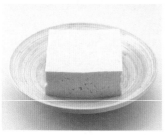

Scientific name and origin: Soybeans are yellow seeds of the Leguminosae family. Latin name: *Glycine max* (L.) Merr. They are found in most provinces of China.

Properties and taste: Neutral; sweet (soybean and soymilk). Cool; sweet (tofu)

Channels of entry: Spleen, stomach and large intestine

Composition and pharmacology: The isoflavones in soy may reduce the risk of breast cancer by binding to estrogen receptor sites in mammary gland cells. Soy's ability to reduce cholesterol has been attributed, at least in part, to the genistein it contains. Soy is effective in reducing the risk of prostate cancer, and has also shown promise in slowing bone loss in postmenopausal osteoporosis. Soy has 6 times the protein of rice, but half as many carbohydrates. Unsweetened soymilk has less than 70 calories per 100ml. It is high in anti-oxidant, anti-bacterial and estrogen-like functions.

Culinary usage and medical applications:
Soybean and soymilk

1. Strengthening the digestive system and moistening dryness: Soy products, especially soybean and soymilk, can strengthen and moisten. They are more useful for chronic and weak cough, chronic diarrhea, etc.

2. Improving digestion: Soymilk can promote weight gain in people who are too thin by improving their digestion.

3. Fighting joint pain: People who have arthritis and joint pain may experience some relief by eating soy products.

Tofu

Clearing away heat: Since gypsum is added to produce tofu, the temperature (as defined by TCM) is cooler than soymilk. Therefore tofu can treat acute eye infection or lung infection showing asthma and cough with green yellow mucus. Tofu will ameliorate conditions in people who have stomach heat with bad breath.

How to eat?

1. Fresh: Eat fresh whole bean (still within the pod) as edamame, or stir-fry shelled beans with other vegetables.

2. Dried: After stir-frying dried soybeans until they become dark yellow, soak them in rice wine. After two weeks, you can drink the wine for aching joints caused by arthritis or child birth, or for calf spasms.

3. Soymilk and tofu: Soy products including soymilk, tofu and protein powder are widely available, and can be used in a variety of ways. Soymilk can replace cow's milk, especially for those who are lactose-intolerant. Drinking 100ml of soymilk or eating 150g of tofu per day will reduce sweating, moisten dry skin, and facilitate sound sleep. Continue for one week.

Contraindication:

People who suffer from gout or high urine acidity should avoid too much tofu.

Do not cook tofu with spinach.

Too much soy can cause gas. Soy should not be combined with other forms of protein or sugar as it reduces the medicinal properties and leads to indigestion.

Take caution that edamame have not been frozen or stored

for too long.

With protein products, especially soy protein powder, be careful not to consume too much or else stones might develop.

Spinach 菠菜

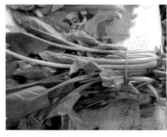

Scientific name and origin: Spinach is an edible flowering plant of the family of Chenopodiaceae. Latin name: *Spinacia oleracea* L. It is native to central and southwestern Asia, but it now grows all over China.

Properties and taste: Neutral to cool; sweet

Channels of entry: Liver, stomach, small and large intestines

Composition and pharmacology: Spinach contains a carotenoid called nexoxanthin, which can cause prostate cancer cells to self-destruct. It contains vitamin K, which helps maintain bone health, while its vitamin E helps slow mental decline and memory loss. Spinach is an excellent source of iron, which is critical for women in menopause and for people who have anemia or chronic fatigue syndrome. The chemical composition includes spinasaponin A and B, and protocatechuic acid, which are thought to have anti-bacterial and anti-mutagenesis properties.

Culinary usage and medical applications:

1. Strengthening the five *zang*-organs: Spinach can prevent and treat headache.

2. Treating abnormally-ascending qi and regulating the digestive system: It helps nausea and gas.

3. Nourishing the blood, arresting bleeding: Spinach stops bleeding include nose bleeds, hemorrhoids and other skin bleeding conditions associated with a vitamin C deficiency.

4. Clearing heat, keeping fluid in the body: Spinach moistens dryness, and it is noted for its work on diabetes symptoms including excessive thirst and chronic constipation.

5. Strengthening the liver and bringing shine to the eyes:

It can strengthen the liver, and it helps conditions resulting in dizziness, irritability, blurred vision or poor night vision.

How to eat?

1. Raw: Organic spinach can be eaten as salad, or mixed with carrots for vegetable juice.

2. Stir-fried: Stir-fry (or sauté) with minced garlic for 2 minutes or with eggs.

3. Soup or hot-pot

4. Boiled or steamed: Cook quickly (do not overcook) to make an appetizer or side dish.

5. Decoction: Use spinach seeds together with wild chrysanthemum to treat cough and asthma or red swelling eyes.

Contraindication:

The oxalate content in spinach binds with calcium, decreasing its absorption; thus spinach should not be eaten with too many calcium-rich products as it may induce stones.

Those who have a weak constitution with loose stool should use caution.

Spring Onion 葱

Scientific name and origin: Spring onion comes from the leaf and stem of a plant of the Liliaceae family, with the Latin name of *Allium fistulosum* L. It grows all over China.

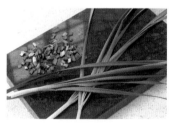

Properties and taste: Warm; spicy

Channels of entry: Lung and stomach

Composition and pharmacology:

Spring onion contains calcium oxalate, alliin lyase, macilage and allicin. Animal tests show that it regulates vascellum muscle movement of the heart, tranquilizes the mind and works against aches. Laboratory research also shows that it works against micro-organisms.

Culinary usage and medical applications:

1. Preventing and limiting conditions: Spring onion opens up sweat pores and regulates the natural function and immunity of your exterior. It is useful for colds and flu, and inhibits the onset of water retention above the chest, as well as cold abdominal pain.

2. Detoxifying: Spring onion removes irritants from mosquito bites, and prevents constipation and reduced urine. It also assists in the early stage of dysentery and acne.

How to eat?

Spring onion can be eaten fresh or dry, raw or cooked.

1. Raw: Chinese people use spring onion, in a small quantity, every day for cooking with vegetables and meat. Fresh and raw spring onion (15–30g) is mostly found sprinkled on top of food or wrapped in a savory pancake.

2. Decoction: Dried stem of spring onion can be boiled as decoction for cold and flu symptoms such as chills, fever and headache. Use 6–9g, and boil less than 5 minutes.

3. External use: You can grind fresh spring onion and use the juice externally.

Contraindication:

People with spontaneous sweating should not take too much.

Spring onion does not go well with honey; this can disturb the stomach and colon, and cause bloating in the abdomen and diarrhea.

Sunflower Seed　向日葵籽

Scientific name and origin: Sunflower seeds are grains of the Compositae family. Latin name: *Helianthus annuus* L. Sunflower seeds are indigenous to North America, but are now grown all over China.

Properties and taste: Neutral; sweet

Channels of entry: Lung and large intestine

Composition and pharmacology: Sunflower seeds contain calcium, magnesium, essential fatty acids and beta carotene.

They fight oxidized fat cells and cell mutation, and have anti-aging properties. They also help resolve blood lipids.

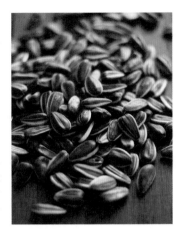

Culinary usage and medical applications:

1. Promoting eruption and drainage: They can help to let out skin rashes completely. Early stage lumps on the ovaries and appendix or joint cysts can be softened and reduced by eating sunflower seeds; likewise they can prevent recurrence.

2. Controlling dysentery: Dysentery suffers benefit from sunflower seeds' ability to stop bloody stool.

How to eat?

1. Raw: When choosing sunflower seeds, raw, unsalted seeds are best. They can be eaten straight or added to yogurt, cereal or salad.

2. Baked: Sunflower seeds are good when used in baking, such as bread or muffins. Or roasted seeds can be eaten as a snack with tea.

3. Stewed: In pork or chicken stews, sunflower seeds add a nice texture, and are especially beneficial for people who have a weak constitution.

Contraindication:

In the presence of acute flu-like symptoms of sore throat and cough, it's best to avoid sunflower seeds, especially salted varieties.

Sweet Potato   甘薯

Scientific name and origin: Sweet potato is a tuberous root of the Dioscoreaceae family. Latin name: *Dioscorea esculenta* (Lour.)

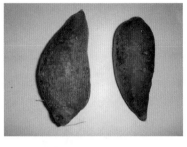

Burkill. Sweet potato is found in Hunan, Guangdong, Guangxi, Hainan and Yunnan provinces.

Properties and taste: Neutral to warm; sweet

Channels of entry: Kidney and spleen

Composition and pharmacology: Sweet potatoes can help stabilize blood sugar levels and reduce insulin resistance. High levels of the anti-oxidants beta-carotene and vitamin C in sweet potatoes may help prevent atherosclerosis, diabetes, heart disease and colon cancer. The anti-inflammatory properties associated with beta-carotene also make sweet potatoes a good choice in the prevention and treatment of arthritis, asthma, fibromyalgia and other inflammatory conditions. It provides fiber to people who cannot readily absorb other vegetable fiber.

Culinary usage and medical applications:

1. Strengthening the spleen and stomach: Sweet potatoes create energy, induce bowel movement, and treat constipation, bloody stool and diarrhea. They also treat burning sensations in the stomach and esophagus. Clinic research shows that sweet potato can treat stomach bleeding caused by irritable ulcers. Sweet potatoes strengthen the yin and qi of the spleen. The functions are similar to Chinese yam, so they can be used interchangeably.

2. Tonifying the kidney: Sweet potatoes also strengthen the yin and qi of the kidney, which reduces dryness and night sweats.

3. Promoting body fluid: Sweet potatoes eliminate lung and stomach heat, and increase body fluid to control dry throat and thirst.

How to eat?

1. Raw: It can be eaten raw, but it is only recommended in small quantities as many people cannot absorb too much.

2. Roasted: There are many ways to cook sweet potatoes. For example, roast sweet potatoes (with the skin on for more nutrients) are delicious for breakfast or a snack on a cold winter day. In fact, they are found at the front gate of many shops in China.

3. Steamed or porridge: Sweet potatoes, either steamed with taro, or cut it into bite-size pieces and mixed with rice for a porridge, are popular staple foods for dinner in autumn and winter.

4. Soup: You can also make sweet potato into soup as you would do with pumpkin. Or peel 500g of sweet potato and boil with 60g brown sugar and water to treat liver infection, especially jaundice.

5. Dried: Slice and dry, then eat as a snack between meals. Dried sweet potato can also be powdered.

6. External use: Powder sweet potato, then make into paste (raw) for external use in treating breast infection. Apply to affected area, then remove when it feels warm.

Contraindication:

Those who have too much stomach acid should use caution.

Do not eat it raw if you have a weak stomach and are averse to cold drinks.

Sweet potato should not be eaten with tomato, as it can induce indigestion and abdominal bloating.

Sword Bean 刀豆

Scientific name and origin: Sword beans are mature seeds of Leguminosae. Latin name: *Canavalia gladiata* (Jacq.) DC. They are mainly grown in China's Jiangsu, Anhui, Sichuan and Hubei provinces.

Properties and taste: Warm; sweet

Channels of entry: Stomach and kidney

Composition and pharmacology: Sword beans contain urease, hemagglutinin, canavanine, amylum, protein and fat. Cardiac function caused by ischemia can be improved by the protein concanavalin A, ribose and adenine found in sword beans. Concanavalin is also thought to prevent tumors. Levo canavanine is believed to hinder the reproduction of the influenza virus.

175

Culinary usage and medical applications:

1. Strengthening the spleen and warming the digestive system: Sword beans can decrease gas and stop yang weakness as manifested by hiccupping. They also treat weakness associated with vomiting clear liquid and non-stop hiccupping, and epigastric distention.

2. Tonifying the kidney: Sword beans can warm the kidney and stimulate yang. They can also be used to reduce aches in the sides of the abdomen as well as hernia and lumbago.

How to eat?

The toxic ingredients in sword beans are saponin, phytohemagglutinin and similar toxins. When cooked at temperatures over 100 °C, these poisonous components can be destroyed. A toxic reaction only occurs when the beans are not cooked long enough or at a high enough temperature. It is strongly advised not to eat raw beans.

1. Stir-fried: Sword beans fried with potatoes is a delicious dish.

2. Salad or filling: Boil and eat sword beans as a salad or use to make a filling for dumplings.

3. Decoction: Boil dried sword beans and their shells as an herbal medicine to regulate qi stagnation or abnormally-ascending qi of the stomach.

4. Powder: First stir-fry the beans, then grind into powder.

Contraindication:

If the beans are eaten raw, or are not cooked long enough, and a toxic reaction occurs, immediately induce vomiting to minimize further reaction, and then seek medical care. Avoid sword beans if you have stomach-heat, or feelings of burning or hunger.

Tangerine (Fruit, Peel and Leaf)
橘子 橘皮 橘叶

Scientific name and origin: Tangerines are mature fruit of the Rutaceae family. Latin name: Citrus reticulata Blanco. Dried mature tangerine peel is called *chen pi* or *ju pi*. Medically, both the peel and leaf are used. In China, tangerines are mainly grown in Sichuan, Zhejiang, Guangdong and Fujian provinces.

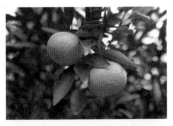

Properties and taste: Warm; sweet and acid (fruit). Warm; bitter and spicy (peel). Neutral; bitter (leaf)

Channels of entry: Spleen and lung (fruit); Stomach, liver and gall-bladder (peel and leaf)

Composition and pharmacology: Tangerine is composed of sitosterol, hesperidin and narirutin. It can reduce susceptibility to some cancers.

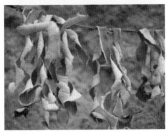

Culinary usage and medical applications:

Fruit

1. Moistening the lung: The fruit nourishes the lung and quenches thirst.

2. Aiding the appetite: It helps lack of appetite and dry mouth, and also helps ease hangovers after excessive drinking.

3. Controlling swelling: The seeds reduce swelling and stop pain, and they can prevent and treat hernias.

Yellow peel

1. Promoting and regulating stomach qi: Fresh or dried yellow peel opens blockages, eliminates pain, and prevents and treats stomach and abdominal distention and pain. It is used in cases of vomiting, diarrhea and gastric disorders causing nausea or regurgitation. It also calms hiccups and belching.

2. Dispelling phlegm and bad taste in the mouth: The bitterness of the peel dries and opens passageways in the body to resolve phlegm, while over the long-term, its spicy nature can dispel bad taste in mouth.

3. Regulating lung qi: Yellow peel is particularly noted for its effect on qi. It balances overactive qi, and prevents and treats hot, blocked qi stuck in the chest, as well as productive cough.

Green peel

Helping the liver system: Green tangerine peel treats liver and gall-bladder illnesses. It reduces fullness and distention, pain on both sides of the ribs, and sting and ache in the breasts.

Leaf

Smoothing liver qi movement: The leaf can prevent fibroma of the breast and treat fibril lumps.

How to eat?

1. Fresh: Tangerines can be eaten as a snack or juiced. Be sure to juice the whole fruit together with seeds and peel, or juice with other fruits and vegetables.

2. Preserved: Tangerine soaked in honey is a good snack. Fruit jam can also be made.

3. Dried: Dried tangerine peel, leaf and seeds boiled in decoction are an herbal medicine to prevent and treat illness. For example, boil dried tangerine leaves 15g, green tangerine peel 15g, tangerine seeds 15g, rice wine 2 tsp and 500ml of water. Drink warm twice a day, a half hour after food. Take for 2 weeks as a course (repeating for 3 courses) to treat fibroma of the breast and early-stage breast cancer.

Contraindication:

During the early stages of a cold, with the symptom of cough with liquid sputum, take tangerine with caution.

Too much tangerine fruit can cause phlegm and sputum to accumulate in the body because its acidity increases phlegm.

Vinegar 醋

Scientific name and origin: While all vinegars have similar properties, rice vinegar is most commonly used in China and therefore is the one referred to below. Zhenjiang city in Jiangsu is particularly noted for its rice vinegar.

Properties and taste: Warm; sour, sweet or bitter (depending on the food from which it is made)

Channels of entry: Liver and stomach

Composition and pharmacology:

Vinegar contains acetic acid, acetoin and tyrosol. Vinegar is thought to have anti-bacterial, anti-virus and anti-parasite properties.

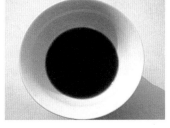

Culinary usage and medical applications:

1. Dissipating blood stasis, arresting bleeding: Vinegar speeds up circulation, reduces blood clumps and clots, and holds blood inside the vessels to prevent bleeding. Mixed with seafood, it can prevent deep vein thrombosis. Vinegar, mixed with olive oil and kelp, is particularly noted for its ability to stop blood clots, including clotting in the brain.

2. Treating abdominal pain, perspiration and weakness: Vinegar works against abdominal pain caused by abdominal masses. It also treats yellowish perspiration (such as in the early stages of jaundice). For dizziness or weakness caused by too much blood loss, such as in post-partum women, vinegar can be added to food to reduce symptoms.

3. Aiding digestion: Vinegar aids digestion in people who have low stomach acid or an atrophied stomach. It stimulates appetite, and dispels water retention and edema. Vinegar can reduce peristalsis of the colon and thereby slow diarrhea.

4. Countering toxins and intestinal parasites: Vinegar counters poisons that may exist in fish, meat and vegetables. Abdominal pain caused by gallbladder roundworm can be eased by drinking vinegar.

5. Treating skin conditions: It can be used against fungus as well as dandruff and itch.

6. Disinfecting and freshening: Vinegar can be boiled and then left in a room to steam out germs, preventing cold and flu germs from spreading. This method is also used as a room freshener. Likewise steamed vinegar can open nasal passages blocked by mucus.

How to eat?

1. Condiment: In Chinese cooking, vinegar is used to prevent noodles from sticking or as a dipping sauce for pot stickers, among many other dishes. Vinegar can also be used in Western cooking or in salad dressings.

2. Soup: Allergy sufferers, with symptoms such as sneezing, runny nose or red eyes, can make a soup with the following ingredients: 5 slices ginger, 12 red dates, 6 tsp vinegar, ¼ cup water and brown sugar to taste (optional). Bring to a boil and continue boiling for 1 minute. Eat when cooled.

3. Drink: To use vinegar for acute hepatitis A, drink 10ml of cooked vinegar 3 times a day. Take for 2 weeks, combining it with a supplement containing multiple B-vitamins.

4. Excipient (medication base): To use vinegar for borderline or early-stage high blood pressure, or high cholesterol, soak 250g peanuts or edamame in it for a week (the longer the better). Eat 3–4 peanuts or beans every night, a half hour before sleep. Take for 7 days as a course, and you will experience effects after 2–3 courses.

5. External use: Soak the affected area in a bowl of vinegar for a total of 24 hours over 3–5 days. If using a concentration higher than 10% (i.e. acetic acid), simply put a few drops on the affected area and wait until it dries. You can use 6% cooking vinegar for dandruff and itch; soak cotton with vinegar and put on the affected area for 5 minutes.

Contraindication:

Eating more than 6 tsp of vinegar per day can damage the teeth and tendons, especially in a person with a damp constitution who suffers from aches, spasms and numbness.

Those with excessive spleen dampness, flaccidity, arthralgia and muscle spasms should have less than 2 tsp per day, or not use vinegar at all.

People who are in the initial stage of infection by virus or germs should take with caution.

Walnut 胡桃肉

Scientific name and origin: Walnuts are kernels of Juglandaceae. Latin name: *Juglans regia* L. Walnuts are grown in all provinces of China.

Properties and taste: Warm; sweet

Channels of entry: Kidney, lung and large intestine

Composition and pharmacology: Walnuts contain fatty acids, including linoleic acid and linolenic acid. Their omega-3 fatty acids promote bone health. Preliminary research shows that walnuts also function against cough. They contain high levels of the amino acid L-arginine I, which is an important agent in controlling high blood pressure. An anti-oxidant called ellagic acid, which is present in walnuts, may block the processes that can lead to cancer.

Culinary usage and medical applications:

1. Strengthening the kidney and warming the lung: As medicine, walnuts are used for asthma and cough, including symptoms of chronic cough, wheezing with shortness of breath, clear or white watery mucus and exercise-induced asthma. These conditions are common in people who have an aversion to cold properties and tastes during seasonal changes, especially children and the elderly.

2. Treating weakness: Walnuts are good for people with weakness in the back or bladder, soreness in the knees, and problems with seminal emission or urinary incontinence.

3. Relieving constipation by moistening: Another function of walnuts is to nourish and moisten the large intestine to treat dry stool, especially when suffering from slow movement of the colon. Similarly, they are suggested for people who experience tightness when passing stool, or who have perspiration and shortness of breath after bowel movements.

How to eat?

1. Powder: After grinding 10g (daily dosage) of walnuts into

181

powder, mix with either rice wine or water daily for 2 months to treat premature whitening of hair or poor memory.

To treat kidney stones and urinary tract stones, use 120g whole walnuts, 120ml black sesame seed oil, and 120g white sugar. Powder the walnuts and mix all the ingredients together. Consume 20g each time, 3 times per day; continue for 6 days.

Women who recently gave birth but have blocked milk ducts can mix 20g of powdered walnuts and 20ml warm water together. Split into two portions and take one portion in the morning and one portion in the afternoon, continuing for three days.

2. Soup: Taking a root vegetable and meat on the bone, bring to a boil and then simmer for 40 minutes. Add walnuts toward the end of the cooking time, just long enough to soften. Each portion should contain 3 whole walnuts.

3. Porridge: Mix 50g powdered whole walnuts, 100g rice (presoaked for 20 minutes) and 300ml of water, then cook for 50 minutes. Eat for breakfast daily for 15 days to strengthen the kidney, and enhance memory and mental acuity.

4. Paste: Crush 10g walnuts and 10g black sesame seeds into powder, then mix with honey to create a paste. Take this dosage daily in the morning for at least one month to treat dry hair and scalp, split ends, premature whitening of the hair, and constipation. The paste can be added to toast, pancakes or noodles, or you can find other creative uses for it.

5. Wine: To treat lower back pain, especially linked with cold and damp weather, soak 9g whole walnuts in 50ml rice wine, then steam together for 10 minutes. Drink the rice wine and eat the walnuts once a day for 5 days. For the weak and elderly, add 3g Chinese white ginseng to the above recipe, steaming it together with the rice wine and walnuts. Note: People suffering from stomach ulcers should not drink rice wine; instead, make tea using 9g whole walnuts, 3g white ginseng and 75ml water. Brew for 10 minutes, then drink the tea and eat the walnuts and ginseng.

Contraindication:

Those suffering from diarrhea are advised not to eat walnuts.

Watermelon 西瓜

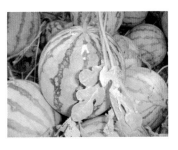

Scientific name and origin: Watermelon belongs to Cucurbitaceae, with the Latin name of *Citrullus lanatus* (Thunb.) In medical applications, both the flesh and the inner rind, as close as possible to the green outer rind, are used. Watermelon is grown all over China.

Properties and taste: Cold; sweet (the inner rind is cooling and sweet)

Channels of entry: Heart, stomach and urinary bladder

Composition and pharmacology: Watermelon is a good source of vitamins A and C, which may reduce the risk of heart disease and colon cancer, as well as relieve symptoms of arthritis and asthma. It can also reduce excessive heat, therefore retaining body fluids. Watermelon has exceptionally high levels of citrulline, an amino acid used to make arginine, which can play a key role in treating erectile dysfunction, high blood pressure, insulin sensitivity and atherosclerosis. The lycopene in watermelon may significantly reduce the risk of developing prostate cancer.

Culinary usage and medical applications:

1. Clearing away summer-heat: Watermelon cools and calms annoyance caused by the heat of summer, while quenching thirst and controlling restlessness. It cures hangovers as it rehydrates and replaces lost electrolytes. It can also reduce the loss of body fluids due to excessive heat.

2. Relieving toxic heat: The cooling nature of watermelon can ease low-grade fever caused by high outdoor temperatures and humidity. In the spring and summer, when people develop seasonal acne or spider veins on their faces, watermelon can counteract these conditions.

3. Inducing diuresis: Watermelon increases urine production and helps difficult urination.

4. Using watermelon externally to treat the mouth and throat: The inner rind is good for cold sores, canker sores and inflammation of the throat. It is also used to alleviate dry and burning sensations in the pharynx and larynx.

183

How to eat?

1. Raw: The fruit can be eaten straight, while the inner rind can also be eaten raw by first soaking it in salt water for 15–20 minutes and then mixing it into salad or eating like carrot sticks with dip.

2. Juice: The fruit of the watermelon can be juiced.

3. Stir-fried: The inner rind can be stir-fried with shelled edamame or other root vegetables.

4. Soup: The inner rind can also be made into soup with shrimp or seaweed such as kelp. With fresh inner rind, use 30–60g per person, or if using dried rind, 10–30g per person.

5. Powder: Powder made from the inner rind is a medical herb for mouth ulcers.

Contraindication:

Due to its cooling nature, people with cold or wet constitutions shouldn't eat too much watermelon. Watermelon should only be used in the summer, as the properties are most impactful and relevant then.

Wine (Rice or Grape) 米酒 葡萄酒

Scientific name and origin: Wine can be made from a variety of fruits, most typically grapes, by adding yeast and gradually fermenting. In China, rice wine is common. It is produced all over China.

Properties and taste: Warm to hot; bitter, sweet and spicy

Channels of entry: All twelve main channels

Composition and pharmacology: Saponins in red (grape) wine may lower cholesterol levels. Red wine may help fight cavities, upper respiratory tract infections and gingivitis. It has anti-microbial properties that fight various disease-causing agents. Wine from grapes contains resveratrol, which may serve as an anti-oxidant. It promotes cardiac and brain micro-circulation of blood. Research shows that red wine can prevent heart and cerebrovascular disease.

Culinary usage and medical applications:

1. Regulating blood circulation: Wine regulates micro-circulation, increases the efficacy of some herbs, and warms the stomach and digestive system.

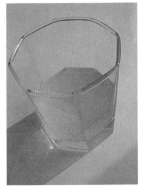

2. Resolving stagnation of qi: Wine prevents pathogenic cold, enlivening the appetite. Wine can treat twitches, spasms, tightness of the chest and abdominal pain, as well as aches, especially those in the arm. On the psychological side, it can sometimes ease people into talking and discussing personal feelings.

3. Promoting longevity and combating disease: Since wine affects all channels of the body and regulates qi and blood movement, it has become a longevity beverage for the aged. There is evidence to suggest that red wine can prevent cardiovascular and cerebrovascular diseases.

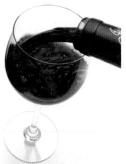

Drinking wine in the right way:

The motto, "no smoking and little alcohol," of the WHO (World Health Organization), means that wine must be drunk in a limited quantity in order to be good for our health. How much should we drink to receive benefits without causing harm to our bodies? For red wine, drink less than 100ml per day; for hard alcohol, less than 5–10ml per day; and for beer, not more than 300ml per day. However, if you don't drink wine, you can receive some similar health benefits by eating grapes (see the Grape section for detailed information).

How to eat?

1. Beverage: To help anemia with dizziness, and palpitation and tiredness, drink 20ml of grape wine 2–3 times a day. In China, wine can be drunk cold or warm (typically it is iced in summer and served warm in winter). Rice wine is better when

warm.

2. Cooking: For extra flavor, wine can be added to meat or seafood while cooking.

3. Decoction: When wine is decocted along with herbs, TCM believes that it guides the herbs (medicine) to the diseased area, especially to the lower back and joints. You can use wine to soak herbs in order to take them orally.

Contraindication:

People with the following conditions should avoid wine: bleeding, dehydration, blood weakness or damp-hot constitution.

Wolfberry 枸杞子

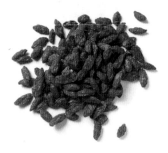

Scientific name and origin: Wolfberry is a mature fruit of Solanaceae. Latin name: *Lycium barbarum* L. It is found in Ningxia, Gansu and Xinjiang of China.

Properties and taste: Neutral; sweet

Channels of entry: Liver, kidney, lung

Composition and pharmacology: Wolfberry contains betaine, wolfberry LBP-I, polysaccharide acid, multi-vitamins and minerals. Research shows that wolfberry can help boost and regulate the immune system. Also, wolfberry helps with iron deficiency and anemia, and can increase white blood cell count. It has anti-cancer properties, reduces high cholesterol, high blood sugar and high blood pressure. Overall it protects the function of the liver and has anti-aging properties.

Culinary usage and medical applications:

1. Strengthening the liver and kidney, nourishing essence: Wolfberry helps nourish and enrich the yin and essence of the liver and kidney. It can help with lower back and knee pain, as well as tinnitus, insomnia, nightmares, spontaneous emission and early onset of aging.

2. Promoting blood products and healthy eyes: It can be used to improve eyesight (near- and far-sightedness) as well as dizziness.

3. Controlling diabetes symptoms: Clinically, wolfberry has also been used to control symptoms such as increased thirst and blood sugar swings.

How to eat?

1. Steamed: Steam the wolfberries, then stir fry with mixed vegetables. They may also be used as a garnish and sprinkled on top of all types of dishes and desserts.

2. Snack: Let the berry soften in your mouth and chew it slowly.

3. Soup: Mix water and wolfberries, using one cup of water for every 10 to 15 berries.

Simmer for 5 minutes, and drink the soup and eat the berries.

4. Tea: Mix 3 bulbs of chrysanthemum flowers with 10 wolfberries in a cup. Pour in hot water, put a lid on and let brew for 5 minutes. Drink while warm. If preferred, the wolfberries can be ground into powder and then mixed with hot water.

5. Porridge: Mix 15g wolfberries, 100g glutinous rice or 50g oats, and 250ml water. Cook for 20 to 30 minutes, and add a bit of honey or jujubes if you want a sweeter flavor.

6. Jelly or pudding: Take 200g wolfberries, 200g dragon eye fruit (longan) and 2000ml water, bring to a boil and then let simmer for 2 hours. Discard the extra liquid and continue to cook on a low heat until all the ingredients have a jelly- or pudding-like consistency. Consume 2 tsp twice daily, morning and night (the above quantity will last about 3 weeks). This jelly is particularly beneficial for nourishing the blood and yin-yang, calming the mind and sharpening memory, and strengthening tendons and bones.

7. Alcohol: Wolfberries mixed with Chinese distilled liquor will make wolfberry wine.

8. Decoction: You can boil the berries with eucommia bark for decoction to treat lumbago.

Contraindication:

People who suffer from diarrhea or are easily prone to developing mucus in the throat and nose should use wolfberry with caution.

Wood Ear (Black Fungus) 黑木耳

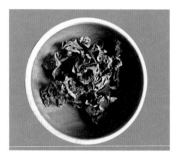

Scientific name and origin: Wood ear is a dry sporocarp of the Auricularaceae family. Latin name: *Auricularia auricular* Underw. Wood ear is found in forests where it grows on dead and decaying wood from oak, pagoda and mulberry trees. It is commonly found in Sichuan, Jiangsu, Fujian and nearby provinces.

Properties and taste: Neutral; sweet

Channels of entry: Spleen, lung, large intestine and liver

Composition and pharmacology: Wood ear contains polysaccharides, ergosterol, protein, fat, lecithin, a variety of vitamins, calcium, phosphorus and iron. Wood ear acts as a blood thinner, has anti-thrombosis properties, and stimulates the immune system. Among other extensive pharmacological effects, it regulates lipid levels, increases resistance to atherosclerosis, reduces excessive blood sugar, helps prevent ulcers, and has anti-aging and anti-fungal properties (for example, fighting candida).

Culinary usage and medical applications:

1. Strengthening qi and nourishing blood: Weakness of qi is characterized by mental and physical fatigue. Those who are pale in the face and lips or who have a yellowish complexion suffer from a deficiency of blood. Deficient qi and blood often indicate an iron deficiency, and therefore these conditions benefit from wood ear's high iron content.

2. Moistening the lung and stomach: Lung weakness manifests as shortness of breath and dry cough, dry throat and mouth. Wood ear can aid these conditions.

3. Arresting bleeding: Wood ear helps replace lost blood and stops further blood loss; examples include coughing up blood, heavy menstruation, hemorrhoids or bloody stool.

4. Relaxing the bowels: Wood ear treats constipation.

5. Reducing borderline high blood pressure: It works on those who have prematurely aged, and is not applicable to serious cases of high blood pressure.

How to eat?

1. Stir-fried: The most common way to eat wood ear is to rehydrate it and then stir-fry with other vegetables or eggs. Soak the wood ear for 30 minutes and clean thoroughly. Chop into bite-sized pieces, if necessary, and then add to any stir-fry or soup. Continue taking for 5 days to ease hemorrhoids and to replace lost blood.

2. Salad: Using cleaned, rehydrated wood ear, boil for 2 minutes, then remove from heat and cool. Mix with vinegar, sesame oil, garlic and chopped chilies (optional) for a spicy crunchy salad. Alternatively, after cooling, add the wood ear to a fresh green salad.

3. Soup: Wood ear is also good made into soup, especially thick soup. It can be added to any kind of soup, such as mushroom or meat soups, in the earlier stages of preparation.

4. Steamed: Steaming is another good way to prepare wood ear. After cleaning and rehydrating for 30 minutes, transfer to a steamer with crystal sugar and fruit, such as pears, for a sweeter way to enjoy wood ear.

Contraindication:

Wood ear should not be eaten with radishes.

Those who have a cold stomach (characterized by discomfort when eating cold foods or drinking cold water) or loose bowels should not eat wood ear.

Chapter Five
Using Functional Foods to Treat Common Health Conditions

I n Chapter Three, we focused on using the theories of Yin-Yang and the Five Elements to explain the properties of individual foods and their effects on different body meridians and constitutions. We also examined circumstances under which to eat these foods, and how to benefit from their abilities to prevent or cure illness.

In this chapter, we will discover the principles behind combining certain foods, using their synergies to help maintain a state of good health. We all experience variations in our health; there are times when our bodies feel less than optimal, with decreased physical or mental vitality. In properly diagnosing your own health, it is important to embrace your life stage and not always compare the present with a healthier, more vital past. At the age of 60, there is no need to try and build the body of a 30-year-old. You have to be realistic about the body's natural development, and pay attention to maintaining the optimal health for your current age. The key is to listen to your own body, and embrace healthy and realistic expectations.

However, modern life can be prematurely aging us. People are "spending" too much of their vitality, draining themselves of it with lack of sleep, inadequate nutrition, and too much stress. The effect of your environment and lifestyle is also important to recognize: high blood pressure at the age of 70 could be a natural phenomenon but at the age of 30, it is an indication that something is causing your system to work less than optimally. The first step to health is to understand what "healthy" means for you.

The WHO finds that 75% of the world's population is in a "quasi-healthy" state, or a state of sub-health or compromised health. This is not only in poverty-stricken populations; in the US, we are seeing an annual increase of 6 million people suffering from lifestyle diseases (chronic fatigue, depression, fibromyalgia, obesity, etc).

In TCM, these states of "sub-health" are considered highly reversible. They are regarded as a turning point, from which people can either return to optimal health or else degenerate into bad health, including serious diseases like cancer, diabetes or organ failure. This book shares methods that will combat this sub-health state, bringing your constitution back into balance using functional foods and herbs that are enjoyable and have almost no side effects.

In this chapter, we will introduce different health imbalances, and present two to three synergistic ingredients that have been proven to achieve the best results. For example, a German researcher, Professor Wagner, identified the synergy that exists between garlic, St. John's wort and the herbal compound berogast. Working together, their multiple compounds affect different physiological systems, having a greater compound effect than each individually would have.

There are two principles that dictate how to pair foods and herbs. One focuses on matching two foods that have a similar function of yin or yang. These form natural and regular pairings, just like the way you might pair red meat with red wine. In TCM, an example would be ginger with brown sugar, or silver fungus with honey or crystal sugar. The second principle is to pair foods that have differing but complimentary effects on the body. This may involve tonifying/strengthening qi or blood through yin and yang properties for the most effective balance. For example, taking ginger (which strengthens yang) and dates (to tonify blood) works to strengthen the body overall.

Through the proper choice of functional foods and herbs we can live a balanced, healthy life, and avoid falling into illness. This stresses the preventative side of TCM, which should be appealing to all: An ounce of prevention is worth a pound of cure!

The following sections offer insight into six key areas of well-being:

1) Getting fit and staying energetic.
2) Enhancing beauty through inner harmony.
3) Regulating and boosting immunity.
4) Maintaining reproductive health and fertility.
5) Reducing toxins and regulating systems.
6) Regulating moods and sharpening mental acuity.

1. Getting Fit and Staying Energetic

Aging is an unavoidable phenomenon. It is characterized by both internal and external changes. On the physical side, there is declined physical ability, weakening of the function of the sense organs, onset of disorders like cardiac problems and diabetes, blood pressure changes and arthritis. There are also changes in appearance such as graying hair, baldness, wrinkles and so on. Mentally, there may be memory loss or a decrease in mental and logical sharpness.

Nobody wants to be old, look old, and feel old, but aging is a reality of life. Every emperor in ancient China looked for special potions of immortality, and the Chinese saying *lao dang yi zhuang* (老当益壮) tells that gaining vigor with age is everyone's hope and wish, and has been for thousands of years.

But the non-stop unbalanced way of living we have created in the modern world makes degeneration and premature aging common in our society. We face problems with the spine, joints and internal organ systems earlier than our age would dictate. Symptoms known as the "three highs" (high cholesterol, high uric acid or blood sugar, and high blood pressure) used to be common only in seniors, but now are often found within middle age groups (without counting those genetically prone to these conditions).

It is impossible to stay young forever. However, by regulating your eating and lifestyle, you can maintain your optimal health. Changing your diet can not only extend your life, but it will make you feel and look younger than your actual age.

And it is not only your physical body that can be improved through functional foods. They can keep you young mentally, maintaining concentration and a sharp mind, and make you feel energetic, strengthening your qi and yang. Toward this end, you should often eat ginseng, astragalus root, walnuts, pistachios, chestnuts, raspberries, cassia fruits, cherries, coconuts, gingko nuts, pumpkin seeds and jasmine tea.

One strategy toward treating premature aging or reducing degeneration is to balance the acidic and alkaline states within the body. Eating more vegetables and fruits can help you achieve a more alkaline state, balancing the acids that build up through unhealthy living.

There is more and more literature citing clinical reports that have proven the efficacy of resolving problems through functional food. For example, there is evidence that vitamins C, E and minerals can result in a lowered risk of disease, in particular of cardiovascular disease, which is a major killer among the developed nations of the world. These can be taken as supplements, but it is much easier and more natural to increase intake of these vitamins by making some easy alterations to diet. By this simple means, it may be possible to substantially improve quality of life, in particular for people of advancing years.

TCM wholeheartedly embraces the concept of using simple plant-based remedies, based on an understanding of one's body type. By knowing your own individual constitution, you can choose the proper functional food to bring about balance, resulting in good health.

In diagnosing patients, I use a rating of stronger (+), average (0), and declining (-) to determine different stages of a condition. The goal of this book is to help you stay at least in the middle of the scale shown below. If you're on the far left side of the scale, don't expect to be able to move all the way to the right side; this may not suit your body type and you may become out of balance again by pushing yourself too far.

-	0	+
Premature aging	Natural state	Longevity

Now, rather than looking at individual foods as we did earlier, we will look at specific conditions of degeneration, examining food remedies that will bring your body back in balance.

Degeneration of Physical Energy and Mental State
1) Imbalance: Mental tiredness, fatigue and sweating (weak type of qi and yin)
Ingredients: 750g chicken, 30g American ginseng
Procedure: Boil in water, then simmer for $1\frac{1}{2}$ hours to make a soup

Usage: 2 times a day (be sure to also eat the solids, i.e. the chicken and ginseng pieces)
Term: Twice a week in the winter, repeating 3 times

2) Imbalance: Mental tiredness, forgetfulness and body weakness (weak type of yin and yang)

Ingredients: 90g black sesame seeds, 90g walnuts, 30g polygonum (Chinese cornbind), 30g dried wolfberries
Procedure: Crush all the ingredients into powder and mix them together
Usage: Twice a day take 3g of the powder. You can take it directly or mix with hot water
Term: Consume the entire quantity created in the recipe above within a span of 45 days in autumn or winter

3) Imbalance: Anemia, pale face, lassitude and fatigue (weak type of qi and blood)

(A) Ingredients: 30g astragalus root, 8 jujubes (Chinese dates)
Procedure: Boil in water, and then simmer a half hour for a decoction
Usage: Drink as a tea, 2 times a day before food (be sure to eat the dates)
Term: 6 weeks
Tip: You can cook a larger batch to last a week by using 180g astragalus root and 48 jujubes
(B) Ingredients: 10g wood ear, 6 jujubes, 1 tsp brown sugar
Procedure: Wash and soak the wood ear in hot water for 10 minutes; clean thoroughly. Chop into bite-sized pieces, if necessary. In a large cooking pot (enamel pot preferred), add wood ear, jujubes and water, and bring to a boil. Then reduce to a simmer for 20 minutes. After 15 minutes, add brown sugar
Usage: Eat as soup
Term: 3 times a week, for 8 weeks

4) Imbalance: Fatigue, thirst, extended postpartum vaginal discharge (weak type of qi and blood)

Ingredients: 15g astragalus root, 3g Chinese angelica root

Procedure: Boil, then simmer a half hour for a decoction. You could also take extract or powder with half of dosage
Usage: Drink liquid twice a day, after food
Term: 6 weeks

5) Imbalance: Vertigo, fatigue and emaciation (weak type of body fluid)
Ingredients: 15g pine nuts, 9g chrysanthemum
Procedure: Roast lightly, grind into a fine powder, and then add honey or maple syrup. Split into 2 portions
Usage: Drink with warm water, twice a day before food
Term: 6 weeks

Degeneration of the Pancreas
1) Imbalance: Diabetes with thirst, easily driven to hunger, blood sugar swings (weak type of qi and body fluid)
Ingredients: 20g astragalus root, 15g wolfberries, dried Chinese yam (optional)
Procedure: Boil and simmer for 30 minutes for a decoction
Usage: Drink as tea, 2 times a day
Term: 1 month

2) Imbalance: Diabetes with thirst, weight loss (weak type of qi with dampness)
Ingredients: 150g pumpkin, 15g Chinese yam
Procedure: Boil and simmer to make a soup
Usage: One bowl twice a day before food
Term: 3 times a week

3) Imbalance: Diabetes with hot flashes, water retention (heat type)
Ingredients: 60g corn silk, 30g pearl barley, 30g mung beans
Procedure: Bring to boil, then simmer for 45 minutes
Usage: Drink the liquid, eat pearl barley and mung beans
Term: 7 days as a course, continuing for 2–3 courses

Degeneration of the Spine and Joints
1) Imbalance: Arthralgia and lumbago in seniors (weakness of

blood with cold type)
Ingredients: 9g Chinese angelica root, 30g Chinese chive seeds
Procedure: Boil, then simmer for half an hour to make a decoction
Usage: This decoction is enough for one day. Split into two portions, taking one in the morning and one in the afternoon
Term: 3 times per week for 2–3 months

2) Imbalance: Lower back pain in cold and humid weather (cold and damp types)
Ingredients: Rice wine, 250g walnuts
Procedure: Let walnuts soak in a glass bottle with rice wine for ten days
Usage: Drink 15–30ml of wine, eat 5 walnuts
Term: 1 month

3) Imbalance: Pain, weakness or sinking feeling in lower back; soreness and weakness of knees (weak type)
Ingredients: 12g fenugreek, 12g polygonum (Chinese cornbind)
Procedure: Boil, then simmer for half an hour for a decoction
Usage: Drink the liquid twice a day after food
Term: 1 month

4) Imbalance: Tendonitis, movements accompanied by soreness and stiffness (weak type of qi and blood)
Ingredients: 100g fresh figs (or 3 dried), 6 eggs
Procedure: Boil eggs together with figs for 15 minutes
Usage: Eat one egg with 1–3 fresh fig fruits a day. Or if using dried figs, boil the egg for 20 minutes and then eat
Term: 6 days

5) Imbalance: Stiffness of neck and shoulder, calf spasm or lower back pain (damp and cold types)
Ingredients: 1 whole papaya, 3g turmeric powder, 2 tsp rice wine
Procedure: Steam all the ingredients for 30 minutes. Divide into two portions
Usage: One portion every night with dinner

Term: 6 days

Degeneration of Blood Vessels

1) Imbalance: Lightheadedness, exhaustion, borderline high blood pressure (weakness of body fluid with blood stagnation)
Ingredients: 9g wolfberries, 9g dried hawthorn berry
Procedure: Add water and make as a tea
Usage: 100ml each time, repeating 3 times a day
Term: 3 months

Case

Malan, a 42-year-old male, had no family history of high blood pressure or high density of blood. However, his annual medical exam showed that his blood pressure was now borderline high, and his blood density was higher than a year ago. He also experienced constant neck and shoulder stiffness and pain, feeling better only for a short while after massage therapy.

He did not like to take Western medicine, so he sought to tackle these problems through diet changes guided by TCM. Since he had body fluid weakness with blood stagnation, I suggested he eat less red meat, only twice a week, 50–75g each time. I also recommended more soy products and oats for plant protein, increased portions of various kinds of mushrooms, and 1–2 cups of wolfberry mix with dried hawthorn berry tea a day. He also received a course of acupuncture treatment.

His neck and shoulder problems ceased after this therapy, and his blood pressure and density got better after 3 months. I recommended that he continue in this course for another 3 months to consolidate his improved health.

2) Imbalance: Hardening arteries, early stage of hyperlipidemia or being overweight (damp-heat type)
Ingredients: 250g soybeans (dried, black or yellow), 300ml vinegar
Procedure: Prepare cleaned organic soybeans and stir-fry for 20 minutes. Wait until they cool down, then put the soybeans into a glass bottle containing vinegar, making sure the vinegar covers the beans. Seal the bottle and let sit for 20 days

Usage: 1 tsp a day before food or between meals
Term: 3 months

Degeneration of Organs

1) Imbalance: Tightness of chest, shortness of breath, neck stiffness, headache (lack of body fluid with stagnation of blood)
Ingredients: 15g wood ear, 30g silver ear, 1 tsp honey
Procedure: Wash and soak the wood ear and the silver ear for 30 minutes. Transfer the fungus (but not the water) to a non-porous steamer. Steam together with honey for 1 hour
Usage: Eat the solids together with the liquid
Term: 3 months

2) Imbalance: Cough and forgetfulness (weak type of body fluid)
Ingredients: 30g wolfberries, 50g silver ear, 1 tsp honey (or 75g crystal sugar)
Procedure: Wash wolfberries. Wash the silver ear and soak for half an hour. Put all the ingredients in a steamer, add 50ml of mineral water and steam for 1 hour
Usage: 20g every day
Term: 2 weeks

3) Imbalance: Fatty liver, rib area discomfort (weak type of qi and yin)
Ingredients: 30g mulberry fruit or seed, 12g Schisandra berries, 15g wolfberries, 1 tsp honey
Procedure: Cook 20 minutes for a decoction
Usage: Drink 50ml, 2–3 times every day
Term: 1 month

4) Imbalance: Degeneration of hearing and tinnitus (weak type of qi and body fluid)
Ingredients: 10g gingko nuts, 15g Schisandra berries, 1 tsp honey
Procedure: Cook 20 minutes to make a soup
Usage: Eat 2–3 times every day (not only the liquid but also the nuts and berries)
Term: 1 month

5) Imbalance: Degeneration of vision and retinal pigment (weak type of blood and body fluid)
Ingredients: 500g mulberry fruit or seed, 500g walnuts, 200g honey
Procedure: Wash mulberries thoroughly, shell the walnuts and crush into powder. Bring to boil, then simmer for an hour. Add honey and stir well, turning mixture into a paste
Usage: 1 tsp, 2 times a day
Term: 2 months

2. Enhancing Beauty through Inner Harmony

Harmonizing the inner body and the outer body is a key principle in obtaining genuine long-term health. A Chinese saying alludes to this necessity: *yi nei yang wai* (以内养外), or nourish the inside so it shines, moisten the outside with care. A beautiful appearance is achievable only if one is truly healthy, inside and out.

In this section, you'll learn how to get smoother, younger, more vibrant skin and hair as well as achieve a healthy weight using ancient wisdom about food and herbal therapy. These remedies are effective for maintaining youth, beauty and a healthy appearance. Furthermore, they allow us to manage our appetite rather than letting our cravings manage us.

In TCM theory, the 12 major channels are frequently referred to as meridians. Every major meridian must correspond to a major organ system (as defined by TCM, not Western medicine). The meridians will also have branches that are less closely linked to other organs. Finally, the meridians will have surface-level lines of energy, including specific points on the skin that are used to manipulate the major organs.

Because of the connection between the organs and surface points along the lines of energy, the entire body, inside and out, comprises one whole system, which moves energy and regulates health. The saying "you are what you eat" implies a one-sided relationship: the food we eat influences our body composition and health. Meridians, however, can go both ways: what we take into our bodies has an effect on outward appearance, while external manipulations on the skin can influence the functioning of internal organs.

In TCM, the external belongs to yang, and can be subdivided into the three yang meridian channels: *taiyang*, *yangming* and *shaoyang*. The internal belongs to yin, and can also be further divided into the three yin meridian channels: *taiyin*, *shaoyin* and *jueyin*.

From head to toe, the body can be divided into three portions, called *san-jiao* (triple energies). The upper portion of *san-jiao* includes the head, upper limbs and chest cavity above the diaphragm, where the heart and the lung are located. The middle portion corresponds to the region below the diaphragm but above the umbilicus, where the stomach and spleen are located. The lower portion is comprised of everything below the umbilicus: functionally, it includes the small and large intestines, liver, kidney, bladder and lower limbs.

Disease typically moves from yang to yin, or from the upper to the lower portion of *san-jiao*. This means it transfers from superficial to deeper levels, and as it does so, it changes from a deficiency to a serious disease.

One way to understand the linkage of inner and outer is to think about the effect of a massage. After a massage, most people don't just feel relaxation in their skin or outer muscles, but have an overall sense of well-being. Manipulating the body's surface energy level is good for the inside of the body as well.

There are many other examples of this linkage: holding premature babies to strengthen their immune systems, energy-healing techniques like Reiki or *wei qi*, the intimate touch between lovers, or even the effect of just hugging someone. Surface contact is well-known to provide multiple levels of healing benefits.

In order to ensure total health and harmony between the outside and inside, we need to use both external approaches (acupressure and acupuncture) and internal approaches (food and herbs). While this book focuses only on food and herbs, we need to keep both approaches in mind. In this way we can regulate our whole system and achieve overall balance.

-	0	+
Appear older than average for age group	Appearance corresponds to actual age	Appear younger than average for age group

Relating to the Skin

1) Imbalance: Dry skin, dull face, wrinkles (weak blood and dry types)
Ingredients: 200g wolfberries, 250g longan fruit
Procedure: Make a jam-like paste
Usage: 1 tsp, twice a day (morning and evening), on an empty stomach
Term: 1 month

2) Imbalance: Dry skin and cracked hands and feet (dry type)
Ingredients: 1 banana, 15 drops of olive oil
Procedure: Mash a banana into puree with a spoon, then add 15 drops of olive oil. Use as a mask to open the pores and remove wrinkles
Usage: 3 times per week
Term: 2 weeks

3) Imbalance: Combination facial skin (dry/oily), facial swelling (mixed damp and dry types)
Ingredients: 15g silver ear, 1 papaya, crystal sugar
Procedure: Wash and soak silver ear for 30 minutes, then boil for 30 minutes (or use pre-cooked canned silver ear). Meanwhile cut papaya neatly in half and remove seeds. When the fungus is ready, add crystal sugar, and put into the hollowed-out papaya halves. Steam for 45 minutes
Usage: Eat as dessert or snack
Term: 3 times a week for 6 weeks

4) Imbalance: Dry skin and constipation (dry type)
Ingredients: Raw sunflower seeds, black sesame seeds

Procedure: Grind into powder
Usage: Eat 1 tsp, twice per day, mixed into yogurt, cereal or other food
Term: 2 weeks

5) Imbalance: Acne, oily skin and uneven skin tone (damp and heat types)
Ingredients: 30g pearl barley, 50g mung beans
Procedure: Make into soup
Usage: 1 cup, twice a day
Term: 5 days

6) Imbalance: Acne, oily skin, redness and feeling hot easily (damp and heat types)
Ingredients: 2 gingko nuts, 10g fresh dandelion leaves
Procedure: Cut into small pieces, and use to knead the skin
Usage: Once every night
Term: 1 week

7) Imbalance: Rosacea, redness and swelling nose (damp and heat types)
Ingredients: 2–3 gingko nuts, 5g fresh gingko leaves
Procedure: Crush gingko nuts and stir with fresh gingko leaves. Rub on affected area and cover with a bandage, leaving on overnight. Remove and clean the nose and face the next morning
Usage: Once every night
Term: 2 weeks

8) Imbalance: Warts on the hand and face (damp type)
Ingredients: 60g pearl barley, 10g wood ear
Procedure: Wash the wood ear, then soak for a half hour. Wash the pearl barley, then soak in 300ml water for 2 hours. Bring ingredients together to a boil, and simmer for 30 minutes
Usage: Eat this soup twice daily
Term: 10 days for maximum effectiveness

9) Imbalance: Dry skin, cold hands (dry and weak types)
Ingredients: 10 lychees, 10 jujubes
Procedure: Eat both fresh in autumn, or boil the dried fruit to

make a soup
Usage: 1–2 times daily
Term: 3 times a week for 2 weeks

Relating to the Eyes

1) Imbalance: Dullness and excess secretion in the eyes (heat type)
Ingredients: 10g cassia seeds, 3g rose buds, 1 tsp honey
Procedure: Make into tea
Usage: 2 times every day in the early morning and afternoon
Term: 1 month

2) Imbalance: Night blindness, blurred vision, headache, tendency to easily lose temper (liver heat type)
Ingredients: 6g wolfberries, 3g chrysanthemum
Procedure: Make into tea
Usage: Divide into 2–3 portions to drink throughout the day
Term: 6 weeks

3) Imbalance: Red and burning eyes with no infection (heat type)
Ingredients: 2g lotus plumule, 1 tsp honey
Procedure: Make into tea
Usage: A half cup each time, twice a day
Term: 5 days

Relating to the Hair

1) Imbalance: Hair loss, premature grey hair (weak type of essence)
Ingredients: 30g black sesame seed powder, 60g fresh mulberry leaves, 30g fresh mulberry fruit
Procedure: Put the fresh mulberry leaves in water. Bring to a boil and then simmer for 20 minutes. Take the leaves out and discard, saving the liquid. Add black sesame powder to the liquid to make a paste. Garnish with the fresh mulberries on top
Usage: Use the recipe above 3 times a week
Term: 6 weeks
Note: If fresh ingredients are not available, you can use dried

ingredients to treat this imbalance using the following recipe: Mix 30g dried mulberry leaf powder, 90g dried mulberry fruit, 350g black sesame seed powder and 250g honey. Roll into small balls (almond-size) and eat one piece every morning and night

2) Imbalance: Dry and dull hair (dry type)
Ingredients: 3 drops of olive oil, 1 drop cider vinegar
Procedure: Add to warm water, and use to rinse hair. Use after shampooing but before conditioning, to ensure soft and shining hair
Usage: Once a week
Term: 3 weeks

3) Imbalance: Premature grey hair, lightheadedness (weak type of blood)
Ingredients: 90g cooked polygonum (Chinese cornbind), 60g Chinese angelica root
Procedure: Grind into a powder or buy extract tablets
Usage: 3g each time, twice a day
Term: 15 days

4) Imbalance: Premature hair whitening, poor memory (weak type)
Ingredients: 250g walnut powder, 250g black sesame seed powder
Procedure: Mix powders evenly
Usage: 1 tsp every morning
Term: 2 months (best to take during winter season)

5) Imbalance: Balding, patchy or rapid hair loss (weak type of qi and blood)
Ingredients: 50g jujubes, 1 egg
Procedure: Wash and boil jujubes for 15 minutes, then add whole egg and boil together for 5 minutes
Usage: Drink the liquid and eat the jujubes and egg once a day, after dinner and before sleep
Term: 2 weeks

6) Imbalance: Patchy hair loss and balding (cold and damp types)
Ingredients: 100g Sichuan pepper, 250ml alcohol (75%)
Procedure: Soak the Sichuan pepper in alcohol for a week
Usage: Use cotton ball to apply liquid to affected area for 1 minute, twice a day
Term: 2 months
Note: If you supplement this treatment by adding 10 drops of warm ginger juice to wash hair twice a week, this will aid efficacy

Relating to Weight Control
1) Imbalance: Overweight or obese with water retention (heat and damp types)
Ingredients: 60g pearl barley, 30g azuki beans
Procedure: Soak azuki beans with barley for 2 hours, bring to boil and then simmer for 30 minutes
Usage: Eat this soup twice a day
Term: 2 weeks

2) Imbalance: Overweight with bloated stomach and abdomen, reduced urine (damp-heat type)
Ingredients: 3g lotus flower, 5g lotus leaf, 1 tsp honey
Procedure: Make a tea
Usage: 2 cups a day
Term: 1 month

Case
I had a client, female, 57 years old, who for the last 6 summers, when the temperature was over 33 degrees Celsius, suffered from stomach and abdominal distention, lack of appetite, scanty urine and weight gain. At night when the temperature dropped, she would then frequently have to urinate, every 2–3 hours. Her energy and mood were down in the summer due to all this discomfort.

Last April, I asked her to drink lotus flower and lotus leaf tea for 2 months before summer started. When the summer arrived, she had no longer had those complaints.

3) Imbalance: Overweight with constipation (heat type)

Ingredients: 150g cabbage or Chinese greens, 15g dried shiitake mushrooms, 2g salt, 1 tsp olive oil

Procedure: Wash and clean shiitakes and cabbage thoroughly. Soak shiitakes in warm water for 10 minutes, then squeeze out water, remove stalks and chop into bite-sized pieces. Stir-fry shiitakes for 1 minute and then add cabbage for 2 minutes

Usage: Divide into 2 portions and eat with lunch and dinner

Term: 5 days

4) Imbalance: Overweight or obese, with acne or lumps, constipation (all types)

Ingredients: Five Element soup—75g radishes, 36g burdock (optional 36g aloe), 60g carrots, 3 medium-sized shiitake mushrooms, 15g radish leaf (optional 15g corn)

Procedure: Use an enamel pot to boil all the ingredients with 2 liters of water, then let simmer for 1 hour

Usage: Eat the solids. Divide the soup into 6 bowls. Drink 2 bowls per day for three days, storing leftover soup in glassware

Term: 2 weeks

5) Imbalance: Rapid weight gain, hardening arteries, borderline high blood lipid levels (heat type)

Ingredients: 10g cassia seeds (or 3g powder), 30g lotus leaf (or 10g powder)

Procedure: Boil to make a decoction

Usage: Divide into 2–3 portions, drinking at intervals throughout the day

Term: 2 months

6) Imbalance: Weak digestion in children, emaciation, anorexia, poor appetite or limited food preferences (cold type)

Ingredients: 10g Dolichos seeds (white hyacinth bean) , 12g dried hawthorn fruit

Procedure: Boil and then simmer 20 minutes to make a soup. Alternatively, make a powder and then mix into any juice beverage

Usage: One dosage per day
Term: 1 month

7) Imbalance: Weak digestion in children, loose stool and difficulty gaining weight (weak type)
Ingredients: 10g Dolichos seeds (white hyacinth bean), 15g Chinese yam (dried)
Procedure: Grind into powder or cook with food
Usage: One dosage per day
Term: 1 month

8) Imbalance: Exhaustion, emaciation, constipation, movable arthralgia (weak and dry types)
Ingredients: 5g pine nuts, 20g peas, 20g carrots
Procedure: Stir-fry peas and carrots first, adding pine nuts 2 minutes before finishing
Usage: Eat 3 times a week
Term: 1 month

3. Regulating and Boosting Immunity

If the immune system is depressed or overly sensitive, it becomes prone to numerous diseases, ranging from the common cold to cancer. The onset of respiratory infection tends to be higher when combined with a sensitive or weakened immune system; in the long-term this can lead to auto-immune and allergy-originating diseases.

Outside influences such as pollution and the effects of rapidly-changing seasons can contribute to a weakening of the immune system, as can internal factors such as anxiety, depression and taking oneself too seriously. This is particularly true in children during exam time or other periods of stress. Allergies have become a worldwide problem and are contributing to a lower quality of life due to ongoing health concerns.

TCM believes that lung qi is our body's defense, preventing illness from invading our bodies. To strengthen lung qi, and ultimately our overall immunity, we need to do breathing exercises and apply acupressure on the lung meridian points, as well as eat healthy foods to balance lung function. In doing so, we can prevent some respiratory illnesses and the onset of allergies.

By learning more about ancient healing techniques, including functional foods and herbs, and how they regulate the body, we can boost our immunity through simple dietary changes and exercises. The scale shown here moves from a weak immune system to a highly-reactive immune system. The best place is in the middle: strong but not over-compensating.

-	0	+
Weak: Allergic diseases, auto immunity	Balanced: Can fight invasive factors and recover quickly	Overactive: Hyperactive qi

Case
Hives and rashes are common complaints these days due to food intolerances.

TCM believes that wind and damp, or wind and heat, invade our body resulting in an internal system that is out of balance.

Tom, 5 years old, was addicted to eating packaged and processed foods such as chips and cookies. Recently, his skin had become very sensitive to pressure. After showering or wearing clothes with an elastic waistband, his skin turned rather red, even swelling.

I first used pumpkin seeds for 5 days to reduce his dampness. Then I used radish stewed with tofu to reduce his wind heat, as well as mung beans and pearl barley soup to dispel damp heat. Tom's skin hives disappeared 2 weeks later.

Weakened Immunity during Cancer Treatment
1) Imbalance: Tired, hoarse voice during chemotherapy or radiotherapy for lung cancer (weak type)
Ingredients: 12g silver ear, 30g astragalus root (2 tsp if using powder), 30g pearl barley, 1 tsp honey (optional)

Procedure: Clean silver ear thoroughly, then soak for 30 minutes. Cook astragalus root with 500ml water for a half hour, then pour off liquid (reserving for later use). Add 500ml water and cook for a second time. Mix second batch of liquid with reserved liquid. Meanwhile prepare a porridge made of silver ear and pearl barley. Once the porridge is ready, mix with the prepared astragalus root liquid. If using astragalus root power, just add it directly to the prepared porridge

Usage: Divide this dosage into 2 portions, eat once in the morning and once in the afternoon. Silver ear in the form of tremella polysaccharide capsules may also be available. Take one capsule while eating the above porridge

Term: Long-term treatment, at least 3 months

2) Imbalance: Dry cough during chemotherapy for lung cancer (dry type)

Ingredients: 10g silver ear, 15g lily bulb (or 1 tsp powder), 1 tsp honey (optional)

Procedure: Wash and soak silver ear in the same manner as above. Then simmer into soup for 20 minutes. If using fresh or dried lily bulbs, simmer together with silver ear. If using power, add powder after 20 minutes

Usage: Divide into 2 portions, eat once in the morning and once in the afternoon

Term: Long-term treatment, at least 3 months

Digestive System Disorders

1) Imbalance: H pylori (+) and bitter taste in the mouth (heat type)

Ingredients: 30g pearl barley, 30g dandelion root or leaves

Procedure: Make into decoction

Usage: Divide into 2 portions, drink twice a day

Term: 2 months

2) Imbalance: Bloated stomach, vomiting phlegm (cold and dry types)

Ingredients: $^1/_2$ tsp ginger juice, 1 tsp honey

Procedure: Make juice from fresh ginger and add honey
Usage: Take above dosage twice a day
Term: 3 days

3) Imbalance: Thirst with ulcers of the stomach, esophagus or mouth (dry and weak types)
Ingredients: 15g silver ear, 15g lotus seeds, 2 tsp honey (optional)
Procedure: Clean silver ear and lotus seeds, and soak for 30 minutes. Simmer for 1 hour to make a soup. When serving, add the honey
Usage: Divide into 2 portions and eat on an empty stomach
Term: 1 week

Cold and Flu
1) Imbalance: Onset of cold or flu, chill, body aches (cold type)
Ingredients: 5g fresh ginger, 3–5g brown sugar
Procedure: Bring water, brown sugar, and ginger to a boil. Drink a large cup while still hot. Go to bed immediately after drinking, covered with lots of blankets to sweat out the cold
Usage: One or two times a day
Term: 2 days
Note: This drink is also a good preventative against the onset of a cold. The same tea, but made with dried ginger or ginger tablets, can also prevent or ease menstrual cramps

2) Imbalance: Cold hands and feet, sensitivity to temperature change (cold type)
Ingredients: 3g ginger, 6 jujubes
Procedure: Make a tea
Usage: 2–3 cups a day
Term: 3 days

3) Imbalance: Common cold with cough and sore throat (heat type)
Ingredients: 5 fresh olives, 450g fresh radish
Procedure: Make juice
Usage: Drink immediately

Term: 3 days

4) Imbalance: Flu with aversion to cold or heat, headache (mixed cold and heat types)

Ingredients: 3g mint, 12g black bean sauce
Procedure: Stir-fry black bean sauce with 150g cabbage or eat with food. The mint can be used to make tea or eaten with salad
Usage: Divide the dosage listed above into 2 portions, eat entire quantity within a day
Term: 2 days

5) Imbalance: Flu with aversion to cold, muscle aches (damp-heat type).

Ingredients: 15g pearl barley, 30g Dolichos seeds, 100g rice
Procedure: Make porridge
Usage: One bowl, twice a day
Term: 5 days

Cough/Chronic Pulmonary Disease

1) Imbalance: Chronic productive cough or asthmatic cough (weak type)

Ingredients: 10g whole walnuts, 3g fresh ginger
Usage: Take together twice daily, morning and night
Term: 2 weeks
Note: For children, you can soak the ginger in honey for 2 days to sweeten it before mixing it with the walnuts

2) Imbalance: Asthma, watery-mucus cough (damp type)

Ingredients: 5g dried ginger, 10g tangerine peel, 10g turmeric
Procedure: To make dried ginger, put fresh ginger out in the sun; it is stronger than fresh ginger. Use with the other ingredients to make a decoction
Usage: Divide into 2 portions, drinking twice a day
Term: 2 weeks

3) Imbalance: Prolonged asthma, dry cough, constipation (weak and dry types)

Ingredients: 50g almonds, 50g walnuts
Procedure: Roast almonds and walnuts lightly, grind into a fine powder. Mix the powders together well
Usage: 1 tsp with hot water, twice a day
Term: 2 weeks

4) Imbalance: Dry cough, vertigo and joint pain (weak and dry types)

Ingredients: 50g pine nuts, 100g walnuts
Procedure: Roast the pine nuts and walnuts lightly, then grind into a fine powder. Mix together well
Usage: 1 tsp with hot water, twice a day after food
Term: 2 weeks

5) Imbalance: Shortness of breath as experienced by smokers (damp-heat type)

Ingredients: 60g almonds, 20g licorice root
Procedure: Roast the almonds lightly and slice the licorice root
Usage: Twice a day, eat 5 almonds and drink 2g licorice root with hot water (or take 2 licorice root capsules)
Term: 1 month

6) Imbalance: Productive cough with wheezing (weak and cold types)

Ingredients: 3g ginger (dried), 3g Schisandra berries
Procedure: Make a decoction or get powder or extract
Usage: Divide in 2 portions, eat after breakfast and dinner
Term: 5 days

7) Imbalance: Persistent dry cough every autumn (weakness of body fluid)

Ingredients: 1 juicy pear, 30–50g honey
Procedure: Wash, peel and core the pear carefully, then add honey to the cavity. Place the pear into a heat-safe ceramic dish. Steam for 30 minutes and then eat pear along with any accumulated liquid
Usage: One pear daily

Term: 3 days
Note: Loquat syrup can be used for soothing the throat like a cough drop

8) Imbalance: Productive cough and asthma (cold and damp types)
Ingredients: $^1/_2$ tsp fresh ginger juice, 1 tsp gingko nut juice
Procedure: Make from fresh ginger and gingko nut, or used dried ones and boil
Usage: $1^1/_2$ tsp each time, twice a day
Term: 5 days

9) Imbalance: Productive cough with wheezing and sinus problems (damp type)
Ingredients: 90g radish seeds, 30g dried ginger
Procedure: Grind both ingredients into powder, mixing well
Usage: 1.5g twice a day
Term: 5 days

Skin Disorders
1) Imbalance: Skin itchiness, eczema (heat and dry type)
Ingredients: 80g fig leaf and fruit (or 30g dried), 80g honeysuckle vines (or 30g dried), 6–10 cups of water (based on size of affected area)
Procedure: Chop fig and honeysuckle, put into water and boil for 15 minutes. Use to soak affected area. You can also use the juice of immature figs and fresh honeysuckle vines, gently massaging it into the affected area
Usage: Two to three times per day
Term: 5 days

2) Imbalance: Uneven skin pigmentation (all types)
Ingredients: 2 fig fruits, 6 cloves of garlic
Procedure: Chop garlic and let it oxidize for 15 minutes, then roast or sauté it with $^1/_2$ tsp of oil for 1 minute. Eat together with the figs
Usage: Once per day

Term: 3 times a week for 2 weeks

3) Imbalance: Urticaria or nettle rash, hives, chronic itchiness (weak type of blood and body fluid)
Ingredients: 9g Chinese angelica root, 18g lily bulb
Procedure: Make a decoction
Usage: Divide into 2 portions, taking 2 times a day
Term: 5 days
Note: You can also take a "four-ingredient pill" (found at TCM pharmacies) with a dose of 3g. Take twice a day, for 3 days

4) Imbalance: Hives and skin rashes (heat type)
Ingredients: 50g radish, 12g shiitake mushroom
Procedure: Boil the radish first for 10 minutes, then add shiitake mushroom. Boil and then simmer for another 5 minutes
Usage: This recipe provides a one-day supply. Eat all at once or divide into 2 portions
Term: 5 days, or 3 times a week for 2 weeks

5) Imbalance: Hives and skin rashes (damp-heat type)
Ingredients: 90g mung beans, 45g pearl barley
Procedure: Wash and soak pearl barley for 2 hours, then boil for a half hour. Add mung beans, boil and then simmer for another 20 minutes
Usage: This makes a 3-day supply, taking $1/3$ daily
Term: 3 days

6) Imbalance: Cold skin rash with runny nose (cold type)
Ingredients: 6g white scallion, 12g black bean sauce
Procedure: Stir-fry scallion and black bean sauce together with 150g cabbage, or eat with other foods
Usage: Divide the above dosage into 2 portions, eat all within a day
Term: 3 days

7) Imbalance: Shingles, including blisters and aching skin (heat type)

Ingredients: 10g chrysanthemum or 10g wild chrysanthemum, 10g honeysuckle, honey (optional)
Procedure: Make into tea
Usage: 2–3 cups a day
Term: 5 days

8) Imbalance: Eczema in children (heat and dry types)
Ingredients: 9g licorice root, 9g honeysuckle
Procedure: Grind into powder. Add to fruit juice, or boil 10 minutes for a hot drink
Usage: 2–3 times a day
Term: 7 days
Note: 60g–100g fresh honeysuckle vines can also be used for this condition. Boil the honeysuckle, and use liquid to soak affected area for 20 minutes. Continue for 5 days as a course

9) Imbalance: Psoriasis or eczema, with cracking skin or skin that flakes off every night (dry type)
Ingredients: 10g flaxseeds, 20g black sesame seed
Procedure: Buy both as oils, or grind seeds into powder to eat with salad or food
Usage: Eat this dosage over the course of a day
Term: 3 weeks

Eye Disorders
1) Imbalance: Red eyes and headache (heat type)
Ingredients: 6g mulberry leaves, 3g chrysanthemum
Procedure: Make a tea
Usage: Twice or three times a day
Term: 2 days

2) Imbalance: Conjunctivitis with red, itchy, swelling and achy eyes (weak and heat types)
Ingredients: 100g spinach, 2 tsp sesame oil
Procedure: Make as a salad
Usage: Divide into 2 portions, eating at lunch and dinner
Term: 1 week

3) Imbalance: Acute conjunctivitis (heat type)
Ingredients: 15g cassia seeds, 9g chrysanthemum
Procedure: Make a decoction
Usage: 1 cup, twice a day
Term: 5 days
Note: In the specific case of conjunctivitis combined with headache, choose small yellow chrysanthemums for additional potency. If capsules or extract are available, follow the recommended dosage on the bottle

4. Maintaining Reproductive Health and Fertility

In TCM, reproductive and sexual health is based on the proper function of the kidney and liver, and their harmonious interactions. In diagnosing and treating conditions, it is important to observe and understand the variations that exist between genders, at different life stages or during changing seasons. Then we can alter our diet appropriately for optimal health.

We have different "life rhythms," from adolescence, through childbearing age to menopause. Improving our healthcare knowledge relating to each of these periods can help reduce discomfort and promote well-being. Simply paying attention and eating the right foods may be enough for everyday good health. Here you will learn not only about treating illness but also about health remedies for long-term use as your body goes through these longer periods of transition.

-	0	+
Disturbance of menstrual cycle; infertility (either sex); early ejaculation/ emission; low or no sexual desire	Conceive 1–2 babies; average sexual desire	Overly regular menstruation or ejaculation; overly fertile; high sexual desire

Case

A couple (wife, 32 years old, and husband, 34 years old) had been trying to get pregnant for two years without success. Both had normal test results, as per Western medical practice. However, a TCM diagnosis showed that the female lacked yang while the male lacked yin.

I recommended that the male take yin-nourishing foods such as apple and mango, as well as desserts with herbal berries (Schisandra berry, wolfberry, avocado). The female was told to consume more yang foods, including nuts and seeds such as walnuts and pistachios. I also recommended taking angelica, ginger and jujube soup three times a week. Two months later, they successfully conceived a child.

Relating to the Menstrual Cycle

1) Imbalance: Irregular menses (weakness and stagnation of blood)

Ingredients: 30g Chinese angelica root, 15g safflower

Procedure: Crush into powder

Usage: Drink as tea by mixing powder with hot water, taking once a day. Or use externally, dressing around the navel with gauze fixed with adhesive tape. Change dressing every day

Term: A week as an injunctive course

2) Imbalance: Irregular menses, early arrival of period, heavy bleeding (heat type)

Ingredients: 8 jujubes, 30g lotus root (fresh or dried)

Procedure: Wash ingredients, then boil together for 20 minutes to make soup

Usage: Drink the liquid when warm, eat the jujubes

Term: 3 days during menstruation, repeat after bleeding has stopped

3) Imbalance: Extended menopausal bleeding (weak type of qi)

Ingredients: 10g wood ear, 15ml rice wine

Procedure: Using a wok, dry stir-fry the wood ear until it turns hard and crumbles into a powder. Mix the powder into the rice

wine and drink
Usage: Twice a day
Term: 5 days

4) Imbalance: Early arrival of period (damp-heat type)
Ingredients: 30g pearl barley, 15g kelp, 20g carrot
Procedure: Wash ingredients, boil pearl barley first (presoaked for 2 hours) for 20 minutes, then add kelp and carrot together for 10 minutes to make soup
Usage: Drink the soup when warm, eat the solids
Term: Twice a week for 3 weeks

5) Imbalance: Scanty menstruation, delayed period (weakness of blood)
Ingredients: 15g dried mulberries, 6g safflower, 9g Chinese angelica root
Procedure: Make a decoction
Usage: Divide into 2 portions, drinking one in the morning and one in the afternoon. Take together with 1 tsp rice wine.
Term: During each menstrual cycle, take for 10 days, starting as soon as period is finished. Repeat for 3 cycles

6) Imbalance: Abdominal pain, excessive blood flood (weak and cold types)
Ingredients: 15g Chinese angelica root, 30g fresh ginger, 500g mutton, 3g spring onion
Procedure: Wash the mutton and cut into pieces. Put angelica root into a gauze bag and tie, then put with the other ingredients into an earthenware pot. Add water to a level of 5cm over mutton. Bring to a boil, and then stew until the mutton is thoroughly done, about an hour
Usage: Eat the mutton and drink the liquid, twice a day
Term: One or two times a week, continuing for 5 weeks

7) Imbalance: Menstrual cramps, feelings of cold (cold type)
Ingredients: 5g dried ginger or ginger tablets, 1 tsp brown sugar
Procedure: Boil, then simmer for 5 minutes
Usage: 150ml, 2–3 times a day
Term: 2 days

8) Imbalance: Dysmenorrhea (menstrual pain) and occasional amenorrhea (absence of period) (blood stagnation)
Ingredients: 12g peach kernel, 6g safflower
Procedure: Wash and soak, then make a decoction
Usage: 150ml in the morning and afternoon
Term: 5 days

9) Imbalance: Intractable dysmenorrhea (weakness and stagnation of blood)
Ingredients: 40g mume fruit, 20g cooked Chinese angelica root
Procedure: Make a decoction
Usage: Split the decoction into 2–3 doses to take over the course of a day
Term: Start a week before your period and stop when period begins. Then repeat before the next period cycle to reinforce the effects

Female Infertility

1) Imbalance: Infertility with delayed menstruation (cold and weak type)
Ingredients: 12g Chinese angelica root, 3g dried ginger, 8 jujubes
Procedure: Boil as sweet soup (add honey at end to taste)
Usage: 100ml twice a day after meal, being sure to eat the jujubes
Term: 3 times a week, 6 weeks as a course

2) Imbalance: Infertility with acne, rough skin, dandruff (weakness and stagnation of blood)
Ingredients: 10g rose buds, 15g Chinese angelica root
Procedure: Wash and then bring to boil. Simmer a half hour, then pour off liquid to drink as tea. Pour boiling water again over solids to make a second or third cup of tea
Usage: 2–3 cups a day
Term: 2 months, starting after menstruation

3) Imbalance: Infertility with vaginal dryness, difficulty falling asleep (heat and dry type)
Ingredients: 3g saffron crocus, 20g silver ear

Procedure: Bring silver ear to boil, then simmer for a half hour. Add saffron crocus and cook for another 5 minutes, eating as a dessert
Usage: Twice a day
Term: 10 days each month, repeating over a course of 3 months

Miscarriage
Imbalance: Early signs of miscarriage (weak qi type)
Ingredients: 20g cooked mume fruit (black plum), 6g prepared licorice root, 30g Chinese yam
Procedure: Make a decoction
Usage: Twice a day
Term: 5 days

Post-partum Conditions
1) Imbalance: Post-partum constipation, extended vaginal discharge (weak type of qi and blood)
Ingredients: 20g dried lychees, 100g oats
Procedure: Cook together to make oatmeal
Usage: Eat for breakfast
Term: One week

2) Imbalance: Aid uterine recovery after giving birth (weakness and stagnation of blood)
Ingredients: 12g Chinese angelica root, 9g peach kernel
Procedure: Make into a decoction
Usage: Divide into 2 portions, taking in the morning and afternoon
Term: 5 days

Problems with Ejaculation/Emission and Male Infertility
1) Imbalance: Weakness of kidney inducing impotence and early ejaculation/emission (weak yin type)
Ingredients: 250g black sesame seeds, 250g Schisandra berries, 300g honey
Procedure: Make a paste (or you may opt to grind into a fine powder)
Usage: 1 tsp, 2 times a day on an empty stomach
Term: 1 month

2) Imbalance: Impotence with aversion to cold (weak and cold type)
Ingredients: 100g Chinese raspberries, 100g chive seeds
Procedure: Make a paste (or grind into a fine powder)
Usage: 1 tsp, 2 times a day on an empty stomach, drinking with warm water
Term: 1 month

3) Imbalance: Male sexual dysfunction or impotence and exhaustion (weak qi type)
Ingredients: 750g chicken, 30 jujubes
Procedure: Boil, then stew for 1 ½ hours to make a soup
Usage: 2 times a day, being sure to also eat the chicken and dates
Term: Twice a week during winter, repeating 3 times

4) Imbalance: Impotence and early ejaculation (cold type)
Ingredients: 500g fresh lychees, 500ml wine (with low alcohol content)
Procedure: Remove lychee skin, then soak in wine for a week to make a fruit wine
Usage: 20ml twice a day and eat some of the lychees
Term: 1 month

5) Imbalance: Frequent urination, seminal emission (weak yang type)
Ingredients: 15g fenugreek, 15g Chinese raspberries
Procedure: Bring to boil, then simmer for 30 minutes to make a decoction
Usage: Mix with warm rice wine, and drink 2 times a day
Term: 2 weeks

6) Imbalance: Low sperm count (weak type of yin)
Ingredients: 5g Schisandra berries, 5g wolfberries, 1 avocado
Procedure: Soften the berries by pouring boiling water over them and letting sit for 5 minutes. Eat them together with avocado
Usage: Once or twice a day between meals
Term: 2 weeks

7) Imbalance: Small quantity of ejaculate (weak type of yin and yang)
Ingredients: 15g mulberries, half a pomegranate, 15g Chinese raspberries
Procedure: If all berries are fresh, make a juice. Otherwise mix with vegetables
Usage: Once or twice a day between meals
Term: 2 weeks

Prostatic Hypertrophy (Enlarged Prostate)
Imbalance: Preventing prostatic hypertrophy (qi weakness with stagnation of blood)
Ingredients: 100g astragalus root, 10g wood ear, 30g kelp
Procedure: Make into soup, cooking for 45 minutes then removing astragalus root
Usage: Take this soup on an empty stomach, being sure to eat the wood ear and kelp
Term: Twice a week, repeating 3 times

Menopause
1) Imbalance: Flushed face, headache, constipation (heat and dry types)
Ingredients: 5g black sesame seeds or 2 tsp sesame oil, 80g spinach
Procedure: Add spinach to boiling water and cook for 2 minutes. Sprinkle sesame on spinach
Usage: Twice a day
Term: 5 days

2) Imbalance: Menopausal hot flashes and sweating, difficulty falling asleep (heat type)
Ingredients: 100g tofu, 50g radish
Procedure: Make a salad of the radishes and uncooked tofu with 1 tsp vinegar and sesame oil. Or boil radishes with tofu and spread chopped spring onion on top when serving
Usage: Divide into 2 servings to eat over the course of a day, or eat entire portion at lunch time

Term: 3 times a week for 2 weeks

3) Imbalance: Menopausal hot flashes, dry skin and constipation (dry type)

Ingredients: 250ml soymilk, 1 tsp flaxseeds
Procedure: Grind flaxseeds into powder and eat with the soy milk
Usage: Daily for breakfast
Term: 1 week

4) Imbalance: Menopause symptoms including uneven pigmentation, osteoporosis (weak and heat type)

Ingredients: 10g American ginseng, 20g polygonum (Chinese cornbind)
Procedure: Boil in water, then simmer for half an hour to make a decoction
Usage: Drink 50ml, 2–3 times every day
Term: 1 month

5. Reducing Toxins and Regulating Systems

Radiation, pollution and chemical-laden foods compromise our health, often making us feel muddy-headed, and causing skin conditions such as acne, or bloating and digestive problems. Therefore, it is a good idea to periodically detoxify our bodies. Functional TCM foods and herbs are rich in anti-oxidants. Using diet strategies based on the TCM techniques learned in this section will allow you to detoxify and feel healthier.

-	0	+
Irregular elimination; accumulated toxicity from stagnation	Smooth elimination, not much obstruction	Able to absorb varied nutrients, strong elimination (urine, stool, sweat and sexual fluids)

Common Foods that Are Rich in Anti-oxidants			
	Neutral	Cool	Warm
Vitamin A & beta-carotene	carrot pumpkin apricot sweet potato	tomato cantaloupe broccoli	kale sweet potato peach
Vitamin C	fig kiwi fruit	orange lemon tomato broccoli blueberry fig	green pepper strawberry
Vitamin E	linseed rye olive oil alfalfa sprout spinach asparagus	buckwheat artichoke asparagus spinach	oats quinoa watercress
Selenium	salmon oyster egg sunflower seed	clam crab chum salmon swordfish tuna	beef mutton lobster chicken garlic

Case

Constipation and internal cysts and lumps have become common conditions. Many people are not in the habit of drinking water, sometimes because they want to reduce their number of trips to the restroom. And our liquid intake is often in the form of coffee, tea, soft drinks or alcohol, which can raise energy levels and happiness, but only briefly.

I had a female patient, Lin, 53 years old, who had suffered from breast cysts and fibroma, enduring 3 surgeries. She also had 2 thyroids cysts and many knots between her muscles and tissues. She did not want to undergo further operations, so she sought help from TCM.

I found that she drank insufficient water because she did not readily feel thirst. She drank water only twice a week, 220ml each time, along with 2 cans of Coca-Cola or Pepsi daily during spring and summer. She only passed stool 2–3 times per week.

Her condition was diagnosed as excess phlegm-blood stagnation, and I recommended she drink 5 cups of water daily: 2 cups of warm water (adding lemon, honey or sea salt if desired) a half hour before breakfast or lunch, and the other three between meals. She was also directed to take 5g of green tea twice a day, and eat vegetable soup 3 times a week. This was to moisten her body, softening lumps and allowing for more frequent bowel movements.

Spontaneous Sweating

1) Imbalance: Spontaneous sweating (heat and weak types)
Ingredients: 30g lotus seeds, 120g oysters
Procedure: Grind lotus seeds into powder and use in making bread. Fry or boil oysters with rice wine and other flavoring to taste
Usage: The above makes a daily dosage
Term: 7 days

2) Imbalance: Spontaneous sweating and night sweating (weakness of qi and body fluid)
Ingredients: 15g oysters, 15g astragalus root
Procedure: Grind shell into powder, or eat oysters (raw or cooked) and drink astragalus root tea
Usage: Two times a day, with or after food
Term: 1 week

3) Imbalance: Spontaneous sweating and aversion to cold (weakness of qi type)
Ingredients: 5g cinnamon stick, 15g astragalus root
Procedure: Make into a decoction
Usage: 100ml, two times a day after food
Term: 1 week

4) Imbalance: Spontaneous sweating and propensity to often catch flu or cold (weak and cold types)
Ingredients: 5g ginger, 8 jujubes, 5g licorice root
Procedure: Make into tea
Usage: 50ml, two times a day after food, being sure to eat the jujubes
Term: 5 days

Frequent Urination
1) Imbalance: Frequent urination, soreness of lower back (weak type)
Ingredients: 10 gingko nuts, 5g walnuts
Procedure: Boil the gingko nuts with the walnuts and add a little sugar. Simmer to make a sweet soup. Alternatively, roast gingko nuts with shell removed, eating no more than 20 per day, along with 3 large pieces of roasted walnut
Usage: Every night after dinner
Term: 10 days

2) Imbalance: Frequent urination and cold legs (weak and cold types)
Ingredients: 12g walnuts, 15ml warm rice wine
Procedure: If the walnuts are raw, roast them with 1g salt
Usage: Take 30 minutes before going to sleep
Term: 5 days

Constipation
1) Imbalance: Constipation with acne, bad taste in the mouth, hot feelings in the body (heat type)
Ingredients: 15–30g cassia seeds, 9g roasted almonds, 1 tsp honey (optional)
Procedure: Make cassia seeds into tea, and eat the roasted almonds. If you prefer, add honey to tea
Usage: 2 cups of tea and 9g almonds per day
Term: 3 days

YOUR GUIDE TO HEALTH WITH FOODS AND HERBS

2) Imbalance: Constipation with thirst (dry type)
Ingredients: 30g black sesame seeds, 9g almonds
Procedure: Grind into powder
Usage: 1 tsp, twice a day. Add 1 tsp of honey for sweetness (optional)
Term: 10 days

3) Imbalance: Constipation and loose flesh in the elderly (weak and dry types)
Ingredients: 5g black sesame seeds, 5g pine nuts
Procedure: Grind into powder
Usage: 1 tsp, twice a day before food
Term: 10 days

Diarrhea

1) Imbalance: With consistent vague pain in the belly, relieved by pressing, and tendency toward warm, loose stool with white or red color (weak and heat types)
Ingredients: 50g Schisandra berry, 30g dandelion leaves
Procedure: Make a decoction, bringing to boil and simmering twice
Usage: 100ml, 3 times a day
Term: While there will usually be improvement in a day or two, it is best to use for 5 days

2) Imbalance: Early morning diarrhea in the elderly (weak type)
Ingredients: 30g Dolichos seeds, 10g Chinese white ginseng
Procedure: Soak for 30 minutes. Bring to boil and simmer for 45 minutes, then repeat
Usage: 100ml, twice per day, in the morning and afternoon
Term: 3 weeks as a course, you can repeat as it is good for long-term use

3) Imbalance: Diarrhea and bloody stool, ulcer with vomiting of blood (heat and weak types)
Ingredients: 50g persimmon, 2 black plums
Procedure: Eat fresh permission and make dried black plum tea

Usage: 2 cups of tea a day, and 1–2 fresh persimmons (or 1 dried)
Term: 3 days

4) Imbalance: Diarrhea and feelings of cold (weak and cold types)
Ingredients: 10g nutmeg, 10g pomegranate peel
Procedure: Boil to make into a decoction
Usage: Twice every day before food
Term: 5 days

5) Imbalance: Diarrhea and dryness (dry type)
Ingredients: 1 apple, 1 tsp apple vinegar
Procedure: Put ingredients in a steamer, and steam for 20 minutes
Usage: Eat the apple and drink the liquid (optional: add honey)
Term: 5 days

6) Imbalance: Diarrhea and tiredness (weak type)
Ingredients: 24 jujubes, 30g lotus seeds, dolichos seeds (optional)
Procedure: Soak 5 hours and then steam for a half hour
Usage: Use as an appetizer, dividing the above quantity over 2 days
Term: 3 days

Stomach and Abdominal Conditions
1) Imbalance: Hiccups, belching, nausea (cold type)
Ingredients: 6g persimmon calyx, 3g clove
Procedure: Boil to make into a decoction
Usage: 50ml, twice a day before food
Term: 1 week

2) Imbalance: Rib and abdominal pain (cold type)
Ingredients: 3g clove, 3g cinnamon
Procedure: Grind into powder
Usage: 1g, twice a day
Term: 3 days

Accumulation of Lumps or Stones
1) Imbalance: Fibroma of breast and early-stage breast cancer

(damp and heat types)
Ingredients: 15g dried green tangerine leaves, 15g dried green tangerine peels, 15g dried tangerine seeds
Procedure: Make a decoction. Drink while warm with 2 tsp rice wine
Usage: Twice a day, a half hour after food
Term: 1 month

2) Imbalance: Breast cyst (damp type with qi stagnation)
Ingredients: 10g oyster shell, 30g tangerine leaves
Procedure: Boil to make into a decoction
Usage: Twice a day
Term: 3 weeks

3) Imbalance: Non-cancerous breast lumps (excess type)
Ingredients: 50g malt, 15g Chinese hawthorn berries
Procedure: Boil to make into a decoction
Usage: Twice a day after food
Term: 3 weeks

4) Imbalance: Small ovarian cysts (cold type with stagnation of phlegm)
Ingredients: 15g kelp, 15g seaweed, 6g fresh fennel
Procedure: Wash and soak the kelp. Chop and stir-fry seaweed and kelp together for 3 minutes in a wok. Then add chopped fresh fennel. Use as a topping for other dishes such as salad and soups, or over rice.
Usage: Once a day
Term: 1 month

5) Imbalance: Small ovarian cysts (cold type with stagnation of blood)
Ingredients: 3g cinnamon stick, 9g peach kernel
Procedure: Make a decoction
Usage: 100ml, twice a day
Term: 1 month

Edema
Imbalance: Reduced urine with edema (wet type)
Ingredients: 90g corn powder, 60g Chinese yam powder
Procedure: Mix powders
Usage: 15g powder with breakfast, and 15g powder with afternoon snack
Term: 5 days

6. Regulating Moods and Sharpening Mental Acuity

The body and mind are deeply and inextricably linked. This relationship, like inter-personal relationships, deepens with interaction. And like symbiotic relationships in nature, there is an ebb and flow. Because of this, it would be completely ineffective to treat only one and not the other.

Knowing your body constitution is essential to selecting the foods that will help you manage your emotions and live a happy, high-quality life. As noted earlier, you can visit www.acherbs. com or use Chapter Two in this book to determine your own constitution. The website has a database summing up clinical experiences by elite TCM doctors, and on the site, it is possible to learn more about foods recommended for specific individual profiles.

Different emotional situations require different food therapies. In order to feel sympathy and have better personal relationships, we need more qi, blood and body fluid. Therefore, we should eat more foods that nurture these, such as bananas, longans, wolfberries, pomegranates, black sesame, nettles, soymilk, unsweetened yogurt, nori (seaweed) and wheat bran.

Other conditions, such as long-term low-grade stress, anxiety and fear, can lead to weak kidney qi. Or they can disturb the harmony between the kidney and the heart, spleen or liver. Therefore, in these situations, functional foods that strengthen the kidney, and establish harmony between the kidney, spleen, heart and liver, are recommended. These foods reduce the symptoms of anxiety and stress, and help with confidence and relaxation.

-	0	+
Body and mind imbalanced; emotional disorder; psychosomatic disease	Experience a full range of emotions with no wild swings and overall happiness	High tolerance to environment and society, physically and mentally

Case

My professional clients often tell me their bodies feel out of order, and that it is hard to maintain balance or harmony between body and soul. Their symptoms often include fatigue, nightmares about failure, loss of values, and feeling like there is no future. In addition, they suffer physical symptoms: aching bones; knotted muscles in the neck, shoulders or back; pain in the upper stomach or in the kidney and heart area; and premature grey hair.

They describe hormones and emotions that are out of control, causing them to cry easily or raise their voice when talking to others. They may also experience a constant sense of pessimism or lack of concentration, motivation and energy, as well unsociability.

They want to get rid of these symptoms and get back to a high quality of life. These symptoms may evolve into a vicious circle, where physical complaints cause emotional problems and vice versa.

TCM doctors advise these kinds of patients to regain their body's energy by having a good breakfast, doing outdoor activities in gentle sunshine, and taking care of their digestive system through strengthening and nourishing functional food.

Nervousness
1) Imbalance: Nervousness with tinnitus (cold and weak types)
Ingredients: 5g Schisandra berries, 5g wolfberries, 10g Chinese angelica root
Procedure: Make a decoction
Usage: 2–3 times throughout the day
Term: 1 week

2) Imbalance: Nervousness with palpitations and light sleep (weak type of qi and blood)

Ingredients: 30g lotus seeds, 30g dried longan fruit, 15 jujubes

Procedure: Add 1.5 cups water, boil and then simmer to make a sweet soup

Usage: Take this quantity throughout the course of one day, on an empty stomach in the morning and between meals

Term: 1 week

Anxiety

1) Imbalance: Palpitations and restlessness (weak type of yin)

Ingredients: 5g dried lychees, 5g wolfberries

Procedure: Make tea, or boil as soup

Usage: Be sure to take the solids as well as the liquid

Term: 5 days

2) Imbalance: Shortness of breath, forgetfulness (weak type of qi)

Ingredients: 6g pistachios, 6g walnuts

Procedure: Eat raw or grind into powder

Usage: If you use powder, take it with food

Term: 5 days

3) Imbalance: Fatigue, poor appetite, dizziness (cold and weak types)

Ingredients: 50g cherries, 50g grapes or 1 cup grape wine

Procedure: If using grapes, juice together with cherries; or add cherries to wine

Usage: The above is a daily dosage

Term: 3 days

Depression

1) Imbalance: Fatigue, decreased interest in social activities (cold type)

Ingredients: 1 orange, 1 apple with core removed, 1 carrot, 2–3 slices of ginger

Procedure: Mix in food processor until smooth, then sprinkle with

233

cinnamon
Usage: Consume immediately
Term: 3 days

2) Imbalance: Tearfulness, restlessness and constipation (heat type)

Ingredients: 2 bananas, 3g chamomile
Procedure: Make chamomile tea
Usage: Eat the banana and drink the tea
Term: 3 days

3) Imbalance: Forgetfulness and abdominal distention (cold and wet types)

Ingredients: 50g fresh or 10g dried longan fruit, 30g fresh or 6g dried hawthorn berries
Procedure: While fresh longan can be eaten raw, fresh hawthorn berries must be prepared with sugar. If using dried fruits, bring to boil and simmer 10 minutes as a soup
Usage: Eat the fresh fruit or the soup
Term: 3 days

Fear

1) Imbalance: Light sleep, poor memory, easily scared (weak and heat types)

Ingredients: 30g lotus seeds, 50g lily bulb, 100g rice
Procedure: Make a porridge (congee)
Usage: Eat a bowl of congee, once in the morning, once at night
Term: 3 days

2) Imbalance: Hallucination, lassitude (weak and cold types)

Ingredients: 3g Schisandra berries, 2g lingzhi mushroom extract, 10g Chinese raspberries
Procedure: Boil Schisandra berries and Chinese raspberries, simmer for 5 minutes, then pour off liquid to drink as tea. Pour boiling water again over solids to make a second or third cup
Usage: 2–3 cups of tea daily. Eat the lingzhi mushroom extract before food on an empty stomach

Term: 3 days

3) Imbalance: Timidity, closing of throat (wet type)

Ingredients: 10g almonds, 12g tangerine peel, 6g Schisandra berries

Procedure: Boil tangerine peel and berries, simmer for 5 minutes, then pour off liquid to drink as tea. Pour boiling water again over solids to make a second or third cup

Usage: Eat almonds and drink the tea, 2–3 cups a day

Term: 5 days

Irritability

1) Imbalance: Palpitations, insomnia (weak type of qi and yin)

Ingredients: 3g American ginseng, 9g lingzhi mushroom

Procedure: Make tea by adding the ginseng and mushroom to 2 cups water, bringing to a boil and then simmering for 20 minutes. Or grind 30g ginseng together with 30g lingzhi mushroom powdered extract

Usage: Drink tea, eating the ginseng root, or take 1g powder each daily with warm water

Term: 1 week

2) Imbalance: Overly excited (hot type)

Ingredients: 5g chamomile, 15g cassia seeds

Procedure: Make into tea

Usage: 2–3 times throughout the day

Term: 5 days

3) Imbalance: Irritability with thirst (hot and wet types)

Ingredients: Juice from ½ lemon, 60g oysters

Procedure: Eat raw oysters with lemon juice. Or if you cook the oysters, you can use other sauces with the lemon juice

Usage: 2 times a week

Term: 2 weeks

Anger

1) Imbalance: Anger with headache (hot type)

Ingredients: 50g lily bulb, 150g celery
Procedure: Stir-fry for 5 minutes
Usage: Eat this quantity as a daily dosage
Term: 3 days

2) Imbalance: Anger with water retention and fatigue (weak and wet types)
Ingredients: 30g azuki bean, 100g glutinous rice
Procedure: Mix with 3 cups water to make porridge
Usage: Eat a bowl, once in the morning, once at night
Term: 3 days

Mood Swings

1) Imbalance: Mood swings, light sleep, confusion (all types)
Ingredients: 10 jujubes, 30g wheat, 10g licorice root
Procedure: Add 3 cups water and boil for 30 minutes, making 1.5 cups decoction
Usage: Divide into two portions, and drink over the course of a day, being sure to eat the jujubes
Term: 2 weeks

2) Imbalance: Moody with dizziness, blurred vision, constipation (weak and dry types)
Ingredients: 10 jujubes, 50g fresh mulberries or 25g dried mulberries, 1 tsp honey (optional)
Procedure: For dried ingredients, add 2 cups water and boil 30 minutes to make soup
Usage: If can get fresh jujubes and mulberries, eat them raw. If only dried are available, take 100ml soup twice a day after food, being sure to eat the jujubes
Term: 2 weeks

3) Imbalance: Moody with fatigue, soft stool and poor circulation (weak and cold types)
Ingredients: 25g Chinese yam, 15g dried longan fruits, 10 jujubes , 100g glutinous rice

Procedure: Add 2–3 cups water and boil 30 minutes to make a dessert porridge
Usage: Add honey to taste and serve warm
Term: 3 times a week

Appendices

To get the most out of this book, you should prepare a few things for your kitchen beforehand. The recipes will seem easier if you have a pre-stocked kitchen, making you more likely to start using the recipes to take charge of your health. While there are a few specialty tools and ingredients, for the most part, these are things every cook should have on hand.

Tools
Apart from a basic array of pots and pans, essentials include: a wok, mortar and pestle, steamer with heat-safe ceramic container, and an ovenproof earthenware pot.

Spices
The most important dried spices to keep in your kitchen are: cinnamon (including cinnamon stick), nutmeg, Sichuan pepper, cloves, fennel and dried anise seeds. Dried spices like these can be kept up to two years and therefore only need be replaced when they are used up.

Fresh ingredients
Remember to pick up fresh spring onion, ginger and garlic whenever you are at the grocery store. Try to purchase ingredients at the local greengrocer, a whole foods or organic store, or at a Chinese grocery. If the fresh ingredients listed in a recipe are not available locally, look for dried, powder or extract forms. These can sometimes even be ordered online. The dosage of these forms

should be half that of the fresh.

Sauces and oils

The following are essential to generating the complex flavors in Chinese cooking and therefore are used for making the soups, stews and other dishes listed in this book: honey, rice wine, oyster sauce, soy sauce, spicy black bean paste, chili sauce, sesame oil, (dark) rice vinegar and apple vinegar. Most of them should be covered and kept in a dry, cool and dark place, where they will last for up to a year.

Cooking Techniques

Decoction

Decoction is primarily used for medicinal herbs, such as roots and bark, although it can have more widespread applications.

Wash all the ingredients thoroughly, chop into small pieces if necessary, and put into a cooking pot. Add cold fresh water at a ratio of 8–10:1 (water to dry ingredients). After soaking for a half hour, place pot on the stove and bring to a boil, reducing heat after 2 minutes to the lowest setting. Herbal decoctions should generally be left on for 30 minutes, although you should follow any specific directions given in a recipe. Fifteen minutes are needed for a small quantity of leaves or flowers or for a recipe for acute flu or cold. For a meat decoction, check the doneness of the meat; one hour is usually required.

When finished, strain the decoction, preserving the liquid. If seeds or other materials pass through the strainer, use a fine strainer, again preserving the liquid. Most herbal decoctions need to be boiled again, reducing heat to low after 2 minutes. In this second round, it should be allowed to simmer for 10 to 20 minutes. Split into multiple portions if necessary, and drink warm.

Fruit Wine

To make a fruit wine, buy Chinese distilled liquor (50%) and the prescribed fruit. Separate the rice wine into two bottles, and add half of the fruit to each bottle. The ratio of wine to fruit should be 2:1. Store for 10 days to 1 month in the dark, after which it will be ready to drink.

Soup

Prepare all the ingredients, washing, soaking and chopping into bite-sized pieces as needed. Put fresh water and ingredients into a large cooking pot (enamel preferred), and bring to a boil. For a meat soup, add ginger and rice wine once boiling. Reduce to a simmer for 20 minutes to an hour depending on ingredients (vegetables will take less time than meat). Add spring onion and any other flavoring 10 minutes before done.

Steaming

In a large pot, add enough water that it won't entirely boil away but not so much that it touches the steaming basket (usually 2 inches will work). Bring to a boil, then place the steaming basket with ingredients spread evenly over the boiling water. Place the lid on the large pot, and don't open, unless necessary.

For vegetables, steam until tender, about 8–15 minutes. For 250g of fish, steam for 10 minutes; with each additional 250g of fish, add 5 minutes of steaming time. For meat, steam for about 20–30 minutes until cooked thoroughly. When the time is up, turn off the burner, but leave the lid on for another few minutes.

A recipe may call for using a heat-safe ceramic or glass container to steam. Take note whether the ceramic container should have a perforated lid or no lid. Then place the lid on the large pot and allow to steam. The typical quantity for ceramic steaming is 25–50g. Steaming ginseng or other roots requires at least 45 minutes to 1 hour.

Paste

When making paste, the total weight of the ingredients should be at least 500–750g, with each item being at least 50g. To make a paste, you will follow the same basic procedure as for a decoction: wash, boil, strain, repeat.

For the first round, the ratio of water to ingredients is 6:1. After the first boiling, strain the liquid and keep it separated. Then add water to the original ingredients, at a 5:1 ratio this time, and boil again. Strain, and add the new liquid to the previous liquid. Then, using a 4:1 ratio, boil, strain and add this to existing liquid, discarding all the solids. Use a cloth strainer and strain the combined liquid once more.

Place the strained liquid in a cooking pot and use medium-low heat to reduce further. Once the water has mostly boiled off and it has become sticky, add honey to taste. Remove from heat and store in a glass or ceramic container in the refrigerator. For most pastes, you will eat 1 tablespoon a day, spreading it on toast or adding to hot water for a syrupy drink.

Porridge

Put water and ingredients in a pot, with a 6:1 ratio of water to ingredients. Bring to a boil, then after 2 minutes, reduce to a simmer. Cover with a lid (with some ventilation, most rice cookers come with a small hole or vent); stir only once. For oats, simmer for 20 minutes. For brown rice, simmer for 40 minutes.

Glossary

Body constitution (constitution profile) 体质
Body constitution is formed before birth but can be influenced by factors after birth. The constitution comprises features of the body's structure and its physiological and psychological functions.

Body fluid 津液
Body fluid in TCM is a general term for all normal liquids in the body. It is one of the essential substances of the human body and vital to maintaining life activities. Body fluid and blood are both derived from the essence of the foods you consume. Body fluid is a component of blood, and the two substances can transform into each other. Thus it is said: "body fluid and blood share the same source."

Chinese herbal medicine 中草药
In China, herbs are the primary therapeutic agent of internal medicine. Of the approximately 1000 herbs utilized today, 500 or so are very commonly used. Rather than being prescribed individually, herbs are usually combined into formulas, containing 2–25 herbs, which are adapted to the specific needs of the patient. As with functional foods, each herb has one or more of the five "tastes" and one of the five "energies" or temperatures (hot, warm, neutral, cool, cold). After the herbalist determines the properties of the patient's body, he or she prescribes a mixture of herbs tailored to balance disharmony. One classic example of Chinese herbal medicine is the use of various mushrooms, like reishi and shiitake, which are currently under intense study by ethnobotanists and medical researchers for their immunity-enhancing properties.

Congenital base of life (congenital foundation) 肾为先天之本
The body's constitution as determined before birth is controlled

by the kidney and its function.

Congenital natural disposition (endowment gift) 先天禀赋
In addition to the kidney, prenatal influences on the constitution include the state of nutrition and other influences on development. The health of the mother during pregnancy has an effect on the constitution.

Dietary (food) therapy 食疗
Dietary recommendations are usually made according to the patient's individual condition in relation to TCM theory. This relates to the "four energies" (hot, warm, cold and cool plus neutral) and "five tastes," which are also important aspects of Chinese herbal medicine. These determine what effects various types of food have on the body. A balanced diet leading to health is achieved when the energies and tastes are in balance. When one gets disease (and is therefore unbalanced), certain formerly routine foods must be avoided or reduced while some new ones must be added to restore balance in the body.

Essence 精
Essence, one of the most valuable components of the human body, consists of two aspects. The first refers to the basic material that forms the viscera, tissues, skin, hair, tendons and muscles. The second refers to the reproductive essence, which comprises not only the individual's own reproductive essence but also the hereditary reproductive essence (i.e. that of the parents). The kidney has the function of preserving and storing essence.

Five emotions 五志
The five emotions are matched with the five *zang*-organs: the heart governs joy, the liver governs anger, the lung governs worry, the spleen governs thinking, and the kidney governs fear.

Five functional physiological systems 五脏系统

These systems each have one of the five *zang*-organs as the center, from which stem internal links with the *fu*-organs. They are further externally connected with the limbs and tissues, the five sense organs and their manifestations.

Kidney-yin and kidney-yang 肾阴肾阳

These are also called the primordial or true yin (true water) and primordial or true yang (true fire). Kidney-yin is the foundation of the yin-fluid of the entire body, moistening and nourishing the tissues and organs. Kidney-yang is the foundation of the body's yang-qi, which has warming functions and promotes the growth of tissues and organs. Therefore kidney-yin and kidney-yang are the source of yin and yang in all other organs.

Meridians and collaterals 经络

Meridians and collaterals are pathways through which qi and blood circulate and through which the viscera and limbs are connected. They allow communication between the upper and lower parts of the body as well as the interior and exterior.

Middle qi 中气

Also called "qi of the middle-energizer," it refers to the qi of the stomach and spleen, although it refers mainly to the qi of the spleen.

Property transformation (transformation according to constitution) 从化

This principle states that the same environment will lead to different outcomes and diseases based on differences in body constitution.

Qi 气

Qi is the most fundamental substance of the human body; it is the energy or life-process that flows in and around all of us.

Qi activity, qi transformation 气机、气化
The movement of qi is called "qi activity." The various changes associated with movements of qi are called "qi transformation."

Source of acquired constitution 后天之本
While the kidney is the congenital foundation of constitution, the spleen is the source of acquired constitution. The spleen system directs food transport and transformation, playing a role in digestion and assimilation of nutrients. These functions play an important role in the formation of qi and blood.

Spirit 神
In TCM theory, the term "spirit" is an abstract concept. In the broad sense, it encompasses the outward activities of life, and refers to the comprehensive whole. This includes the vitality of the body, appearance, complexion, expression of the eyes, speech, responsiveness, etc. In the narrow sense, spirit is a collective term for cognition, consciousness and other mental activities.

Triple-jiao 三焦
Triple-jiao is the collective term for the three sections of the body, known as the upper, middle, and lower jiao. It is one of the six *fu*-organs.

Twelve meridians 十二经脉
The "regular meridians" have twelve branches, including the three yin meridians and the three yang meridians of the hands and the feet. These are the main pathways through which qi and blood circulate. The twelve regular meridians have designated origination and termination points, and they circulate in defined courses and sequences. They follow rules in their distribution over

and through the trunk and limbs, and they pertain to and connect directly with specific internal organs.

Twelve units 十二时辰

The day is broken down into two-hour periods, each related to specific organs, meridians, functions and recommended behaviors.

Chou (1–3 a.m.): The liver meridian is on duty to dispel toxins and produce fresh new blood in liver.

Yin (3–5 a.m.): The lung meridian distributes the energy and blood produced by the liver to the organs.

Mao (5–7 a.m.): During these two hours, one should sit next to a window in the light, drink a cup of warm water (rather than tea) and comb the hair and head repeatedly. This helps dispel pathogenic energies in the body and clear the eyesight and the mind. It is also the time to wash.

Chen (7–9 a.m.): This is the time for breakfast since the stomach meridian is active. With sufficient yang energy from food, the spleen then turns nutrients into energy and leaves no extra fat to accumulate (if one doesn't overeat).

Si (9–11 a.m.): Blood and energy flow to the spleen meridian supporting metabolism. Nutrients are converted into blood and energy, and sent to the muscles. This is a prime time for working since the energy and blood distributed by the spleen will support activity.

Wu (11–1 p.m.): A balanced, nutritious lunch is important; it shouldn't be too big. Take a slow walk after lunch and rub the stomach and lower back to get the spleen and kidney active. Drinking a little tea and taking a half hour's nap is recommended.

Wei (1–3 p.m.): After lunch and a nap (no more than an hour), it is time for more activity, as the small intestine works to separate and distribute digested nutrients.

Shen (3–5 p.m.): The two bladder meridians go to work, one on each side of the spine, running from the foot to the head. Since energy and blood flow into the brain, it is a good time for efficient work and study. Afternoon tea is recommended. The bladder meridian is also a major toxin-expelling channel and handles toxins dispelled by other meridians. Drinking extra water allows toxins to be passed in urine.

You (5–7 p.m.): The kidneys start to store "essence" as the kidney meridian takes its turn. This is the best time for kidney-reinforcing therapy. It's time for dinner but not too much. A little wine is good to activate blood circulation.

Xu (7–9 p.m.): The pericardium is the fluid-filled sac that surrounds the heart and the roots of major blood vessels. It contains channels of blood and energy. When it is activated at xu, it dispels all the pathogenic energy around the heart to protect it. At this time it's advised to soak the feet in hot water, which can help dispel pathogenic heat and damp, activating blood circulation. Massaging the yong quan point (the arch of foot) in both feet can help nourish kidney energy.

Hai (9–11 p.m.) and Zi (11 p.m.–1 a.m.): Zi is the darkest hour when strong yin energy starts to fade and yang energy begins to grow. Sufficient yang energy allows people to stay active during the day, so it should be well-stored at the right time. Since sleep is the best way to store yang energy, it is best to be in deep sleep at zi, which means you should go to sleep at hai. People should not go outdoors from hai to zi. Hai is also the best time of the day for sex (also for getting pregnant), when yin and yang are in balance in the body and in the universe.

Yin-yang 阴阳

Yin and yang are the two fundamental principles or forces in the universe, opposing and supplementing each other. Yin includes blood, body fluid and visible material; yang includes qi, the functions of the body, and invisible material.

Zang-fu organs 脏腑

The internal organs of the human body are called the *zang-fu* organs.

Five *zang*-organs (五脏): The heart, lung, spleen, liver and kidney are known as the five *zang*-organs.

Six *fu*-organs (六腑): The gallbladder, stomach, small intestine, large intestine, urinary bladder and triple-jiao are called the six-*fu* organs.

Extraordinary *fu*-organs (奇恒之腑): Called "qiheng", denoting extraordinary, these are the brain, marrow, bone, blood vessels, gallbladder and uterus.

Relationship between *zang-fu* organs (脏腑表里关系): "*Zang*" pertains to yin while "*fu*" pertains to yang. Therefore, the relationships between the *zang*-organs and the *fu*-organs refer to yin-yang and exterior-interior relationships.

Bibliography

English

Beijing University of Traditional Chinese Medicine. *Basic Theories of Traditional Chinese Medicine*. Beijing: Academy Press, 1998.

Cheng, Xinnong. *Chinese Acupuncture and Moxibustion*. Beijing: Foreign Languages Press, 1987.

Leggett, Daverick. *Helping Ourselves: A Guide to Traditional Chinese Food Energetics*. England: Meridian Press, 1994.

Maciocia, Giovanni. *The Foundations of Chinese Medicine*. London: Churchill Livingstone, 1989.

Mitchell, Deborah. *The Complete Book of Nutritional Healing*. New York: St. Martin's Press, 2009.

Peterson, Nicola. *Herbs and Health*. London: Bloomsbury Books, 1993.

Wiseman, Nigel, and Andrew Ellis. *Fundamentals of Chinese Medicine*. rev. ed. Massachusetts: Paradigm Publications, 1996.

Yellow Emperor Chinese Classics (Chinese-English). Modern Chinese translation by Zhang Chun, English translation by Feng Yu, explanation and annotation by Yu Mingguang. Hunan: Yuelu Publishing House, 2006.

Zhang, Enqin, and Shi, Lanhua, eds. *Basic Theory of Traditional Chinese Medicine*. Shanghai: Publishing House of Shanghai College of Traditional Chinese Medicine, 1990.

Zhang, Enqin, and Zhang, Wengao, eds. *Chinese Medicated Diet*. Shanghai: Publishing House of Shanghai College of Traditional Chinese Medicine, 1990.

Zhang, Qian. "The TCM Body Clock." *Shanghai Daily*, December 21, 2010.

Zhang, Yifang. *Using Traditional Chinese Medicine to Manage Your Emotional Health*. New York: Better Link Press, 2013.

Zuo, Yanfu, and Tang, Decai. *Science of Chinese Materia Medica*. Shanghai: Publishing House of Shanghai University of Traditional Chinese Medicine, 2003.

Zuo, Yanfu, and Wu, Changguo. *Basic Theory of Traditional Chinese Medicine*. Shanghai: Publishing House of Shanghai University of Traditional Chinese Medicine, 2003.

Chinese

[1] 陈士林，等．中草药大典 [M]．北京：军事医学科学出版社，2006 年．

[2] 陈伟，等．方剂学 [M]．上海：上海中医学院出版社，1993 年．

[3] 窦国祥．饮食治疗指南 [M]．南京：江苏科学技术出版社，1981 年．

[4] 湖北中医学院编委会．汉英中医药分类词典 [M]．北京：科学出版社，1996 年．

[5] 匡调元．人体体质学—理论应用和发展 [M]．上海：上海中医学院出版社，1991 年．

[6] 南京中医学院．中医内科临症备要 [M]．南京:江苏省科学技术出版社，1984 年．

[7] 南京中医学院中医系．黄帝内经灵枢译释 [M]．上海：上海科学技术出版社，1986 年．

[8] 南京中医药大学．中药大辞典 [M]．上海：上海科学技术出版社，2006 年．

[9] 彭铭泉．大众药膳煲 [M]．四川：四川科学技术出版社，1995 年．

[10] 唐传核．植物功能性食品 [M]．北京：化学工业出版社，2004 年．

[11] 张继泽，等．张泽生医案医话集 [M]．南京：江苏科学技术出版社，1981 年．

[12] 张杰．胃肠病药膳良方 [M]．北京：人民卫生出版社，2002 年．

[13] 张挹芳．中医藏象学 [M]．北京:中国协和医科大学出版社，2004 年．

[14] 张挹芳．孟河传人张泽生张继泽中医承启集 [M]．南京：东南大学出版社，2010 年．

[15] 朱义豪．实用中医养生 [M]．海口：南方出版社，2001 年．

Index